Geriatrics

Editor

DANELLE CAYEA

MEDICAL CLINICS
OF NORTH AMERICA

www.medical.theclinics.com

Consulting Editor
JACK ENDE

September 2020 • Volume 104 • Number 5

ELSEVIER

1600 John F. Kennedy Boulevard • Suite 1800 • Philadelphia, Pennsylvania, 19103-2899

http://www.theclinics.com

MEDICAL CLINICS OF NORTH AMERICA Volume 104, Number 5
September 2020 ISSN 0025-7125, ISBN-13: 978-0-323-77722-3

Editor: Katerina Heidhausen
Developmental Editor: Nick Henderson

Medical Clinics of North America (ISSN 0025-7125) is published bimonthly by Elsevier Inc., 360 Park Avenue South, New York, NY 10010-1710. Months of publication are January, March, May, July, September, and November. Business and editorial offices: 1600 John F. Kennedy Boulevard, Suite 1800, Philadelphia, PA 19103-2899. Periodicals postage paid at New York, NY, and additional mailing offices. Subscription prices are USD $295.00 per year (US individuals), $654.00 per year (US institutions), $100.00 per year (US Students), $353.00 per year (Canadian individuals), $850.00 per year (Canadian institutions), $200.00 per year for (foreign students), $100.00 per year for (Canadian students), $422.00 per year (foreign individuals), and $850.00 per year (foreign institutions). To receive student/resident rate, orders must be accompanied by name of affiliated institution, date of term, and the signature of program/residency coordinator on institution letterhead. Orders will be billed at individual rate until proof of status is received. Foreign air speed delivery is included in all Clinics' subscription prices. All prices are subject to change without notice. **POSTMASTER:** Send address changes to *Medical Clinics of North America*, Elsevier Health Sciences Division, Subscription Customer Service, 3251 Riverport Lane, Maryland Heights, MO 63043. **Customer Service: Telephone: 1-800-654-2452** (U.S. and Canada); **1-314-447-8871** (outside U.S. and Canada). **Fax: 314-447-8029. E-mail: journalscustomerserviceusa@elsevier.com** (for print support); **journalsonlinesupport-usa@elsevier.com** (for online support).

Reprints. For copies of 100 or more of articles in this publication, please contact the Commercial Reprints Department, Elsevier Inc., 360 Park Avenue South, New York, NY 10010-1710. Tel.: 212-633-3874; Fax: 212-633-3820; E-mail: reprints@elsevier.com.

Medical Clinics of North America is also published in Spanish by McGraw-Hill Interamericana Editores S. A., P.O. Box 5-237, 06500 Mexico, D.F., Mexico.

Medical Clinics of North America is covered in *MEDLINE/PubMed (Index Medicus), Current Contents, ASCA, Excerpta Medica, Science Citation Index,* and *ISI/BIOMED.*

PROGRAM OBJECTIVE

The goal of the *Medical Clinics of North America* is to keep practicing physicians up to date with current clinical practice by providing timely articles reviewing the state of the art in patient care.

TARGET AUDIENCE

All practicing physicians and other healthcare professionals.

LEARNING OBJECTIVES

Upon completion of this activity, participants will be able to:
1. Review the impact on the health and wellbeing of older adults who delay care or receive only telehealth care during the pandemic.
2. Explain the meta-skills and knowledge needed to provide excellent care to older adults including an approach to prescribing and de-prescribing, identifying and discussing goals of care, and assessing safety and independence.
3. Discuss the challenges encountered by older adults during the coronavirus pandemic such as accessing digital healthcare, isolation and loneliness, and increased risks associated with SARS-COV2 virus.

ACCREDITATION

The Elsevier Office of Continuing Medical Education (EOCME) is accredited by the Accreditation Council for Continuing Medical Education (ACCME) to provide continuing medical education for physicians.

The EOCME designates this journal-based CME activity for a maximum of 12 *AMA PRA Category 1 Credit*(s)™. Physicians should claim only the credit commensurate with the extent of their participation in the activity.

All other healthcare professionals requesting continuing education credit for this enduring material will be issued a certificate of participation.

DISCLOSURE OF CONFLICTS OF INTEREST

The EOCME assesses conflict of interest with its instructors, faculty, planners, and other individuals who are in a position to control the content of CME activities. All relevant conflicts of interest that are identified are thoroughly vetted by EOCME for fair balance, scientific objectivity, and patient care recommendations. EOCME is committed to providing its learners with CME activities that promote improvements or quality in healthcare and not a specific proprietary business or a commercial interest.

The planning committee, staff, authors and editors listed below have identified no financial relationships or relationships to products or devices they or their spouse/life partner have with commercial interest related to the content of this CME activity:

Colleen M. Casey, PhD, ANP-BC; Jamie Caulley, DPT; Danelle Cayea, MD, MS; Colleen Christmas, MD, FACP; Amber Comer, JD, PhD; Meenakshi Dagar, MD; Jack Ende, MD, MACP; Lyle Fettig, MD; Thomas E. Finucane, MD; Mariana R. Gonzalez, MD, MPH; Chitra Hamilton, MD; Katerina Heidhausen; Nick Henderson; Catherine Bree Johnston, MD, MPH; Teresa S. Jones, MD; Jason Karlawish, MD; Marilu Kelly, MSN, RN, CNE, CHCP; Julie Lutz, PhD; Una E. Makris, MD, MSc; Zara Manuelyan, MD; Lauren McCollum, MD; Alyson R. Michener, MD; Rachel K. Miller, MD; John T. Moore, MD; Keila Siomara Muniz, MD; Elizabeth A. Phelan, MD; Vassiliki Pravodelov, MD; Thomas N. Robinson, MD; Mattan Schuchman, MD; Ellen Stein, MD; Jeyanthi Surendrakumar; Alexia M. Torke, MD, MS Ed; Kimberly A. Van Orden, PhD; Hannah Ward, MD; Travis P. Welsh, MD; Ailing Eileen Yang, BA.

UNAPPROVED/OFF-LABEL USE DISCLOSURE

The EOCME requires CME faculty to disclose to the participants;
1. When products or procedures being discussed are off-label, unlabelled, experimental, and/or investigational (not US Food and Drug Administration [FDA] approved); and
2. Any limitations on the information presented, such as data that are preliminary or that represent ongoing research, interim analyses, and/or unsupported opinions. Faculty may discuss information about pharmaceutical agents that is outside of FDA-approved labelling. This information is intended solely for CME and is not intended to promote off-label use of these medications. If you have any questions, contact the medical affairs department of the manufacturer for the most recent prescribing information.

TO ENROLL

To enroll in the *Medical Clinics of North America* Continuing Medical Education program, call customer service at 1-800-654-2452 or sign up online at http://www.theclinics.com/home/cme. The CME program is available to subscribers for an additional annual fee of USD 300.00.

METHOD OF PARTICIPATION

In order to claim credit, participants must complete the following;

1. Complete enrolment as indicated above.
2. Read the activity.
3. Complete the CME Test and Evaluation. Participants must achieve a score of 70% on the test. All CME Tests and Evaluations must be completed online.

CME INQUIRIES/SPECIAL NEEDS

For all CME inquiries or special needs, please contact elsevierCME@elsevier.com.

MEDICAL CLINICS OF NORTH AMERICA

FORTHCOMING ISSUES

November 2020
Cancer Prevention and Screening
Robert A. Smith and Kevin Oeffinger,
Editors

January 2021
Common Symptoms in Outpatient Practice
Lia S. Logio, *Editor*

March 2021
Rheumatology
Brian Mandell, *Editor*

RECENT ISSUES

July 2020
Update in Hospital Medicine
Andrew Dunn, *Editor*

May 2020
Palliative Care
Eric Widera, *Editor*

March 2020
Physical Medicine and Rehabilitation: An Update for Internists
David A. Lenrow, *Editor*

SERIES OF RELATED INTEREST

Clinics in Geriatric Medicine
https://www.geriatric.theclinics.com/
Primary Care: Clinics in Office Practice
https://www.primarycare.theclinics.com/

Contributors

CONSULTING EDITOR

JACK ENDE, MD, MACP
Department of Medicine, Perelman School of Medicine, University of Pennsylvania, Philadelphia, Pennsylvania

EDITOR

DANELLE CAYEA, MD, MS
Associate Professor, Department of Medicine, Johns Hopkins School of Medicine, Director, Daniel and Jeanette Hendin Schapiro Geriatrics Medical Education Center, Baltimore, Maryland

AUTHORS

COLLEEN M. CASEY, PhD, ANP-BC
Associate Clinical Director, Senior Health Program, Providence Health & Services, Portland, Oregon

JAMIE CAULLEY, DPT
Clinical Advancement Lead in Fall Prevention/Senior Health Clinical Liaison, Senior Health Program, Providence Health & Services, Portland, Oregon

COLLEEN CHRISTMAS, MD, FACP
Associate Professor of Medicine, Division of Geriatric Medicine and Gerontology, Johns Hopkins School of Medicine, Baltimore, Maryland

AMBER COMER, JD, PhD
Assistant Professor, School of Health and Human Sciences, Indiana University, Indianapolis, Indiana

MEENAKSHI DAGAR, MD
Division of Geriatrics, General Internal Medicine, and Palliative Medicine, Assistant Professor, Department of Medicine, University of Arizona College of Medicine, Banner University Medical Center, Tucson, Arizona

LYLE FETTIG, MD
Assistant Clinical Professor, Division of General Medicine and Geriatrics, Palliative Care, Indiana University School of Medicine, Eskenazi Health, Indianapolis, Indiana

THOMAS E. FINUCANE, MD
Senior Lecturer, Part-Time, Harvard Medical School, Massachusetts General Hospital, Boston, Massachusetts

MARIANA R. GONZALEZ, MD, MPH
Geriatrics Fellow, Division of Geriatrics, University of Pennsylvania, Philadelphia, Pennsylvania

CHITRA HAMILTON, MD
Fellow, Division of Geriatric Medicine and Gerontology, Johns Hopkins School of Medicine, Baltimore, Maryland

CATHERINE BREE JOHNSTON, MD, MPH
Division of Geriatrics, General Internal Medicine, and Palliative Medicine, Professor, Department of Medicine, University of Arizona College of Medicine, Banner University Medical Center, Tucson, Arizona

TERESA S. JONES, MD
Assistant Professor, Department of Surgery, Rocky Mountain Regional Veterans Affairs Medical Center, Geriatric Research Education and Clinical Center (GRECC) VA Eastern Colorado Health Care System, University of Colorado School of Medicine, Aurora, Colorado

JASON KARLAWISH, MD
Ralston House, Professor of Medicine, Medical Ethics, and Health Policy, Division of Geriatrics, Penn Memory Center, University of Pennsylvania, Philadelphia, Pennsylvania

JULIE LUTZ, PhD
Postdoctoral Fellow, Department of Psychiatry, University of Rochester Medical Center, Center for the Study and Prevention of Suicide, Rochester, New York

UNA E. MAKRIS, MD, MSc
Associate Professor, Department of Internal Medicine, UT Southwestern Medical Center, Medical Service, VA North Texas Health Care System, Dallas, Texas

ZARA MANUELYAN, MD
Department of Gastroenterology, Johns Hopkins School of Medicine, Baltimore, Maryland

LAUREN McCOLLUM, MD
Cognitive Neurology Fellow, University of Pennsylvania, Ralston House, Penn Memory Center, Philadelphia, Pennsylvania

ALYSON R. MICHENER, MD
Assistant Professor of Clinical Medicine, Division of Geriatrics, University of Pennsylvania, Philadelphia, Pennsylvania

RACHEL K. MILLER, MD, MsEd
Associate Professor of Clinical Medicine, Director of Education, Division of Geriatrics, University of Pennsylvania, Philadelphia, Pennsylvania

JOHN T. MOORE, MD
Assistant Professor, Department of Surgery, Rocky Mountain Regional Veterans Affairs Medical Center, VA Eastern Colorado Health Care System, University of Colorado School of Medicine, Aurora, Colorado

KEILA SIOMARA MUÑIZ, MD
Department of Gynecology and Obstetrics, Johns Hopkins School of Medicine, Baltimore, Maryland

ELIZABETH A. PHELAN, MD, MS
Department of Medicine, Division of Gerontology and Geriatric Medicine, University of Washington, Harborview Medical Center, Seattle, Washington

VASSILIKI PRAVODELOV, MD
Instructor of Medicine, Section of Geriatrics, Department of Medicine, Boston University School of Medicine, Physician, Boston Medical Center, Boston, Massachusetts

THOMAS N. ROBINSON, MD
Professor and Chief of Surgery, Rocky Mountain Regional Medical Center Veterans Affairs Medical Center, University of Colorado School of Medicine, Aurora, Colorado

MATTAN SCHUCHMAN, MD
Assistant Professor of Medicine, Division of Geriatric Medicine and Gerontology, Johns Hopkins School of Medicine, Baltimore, Maryland

ELLEN STEIN, MD
Department of Gastroenterology, Johns Hopkins School of Medicine, Baltimore, Maryland

ALEXIA M. TORKE, MD, MS
Associate Professor, Division of General Medicine and Geriatrics, Indiana University School of Medicine, Indiana University Center for Aging Research, Regenstrief Institute, Incorporated, Indianapolis, Indiana

KIMBERLY A. VAN ORDEN, PhD
Associate Professor, Department of Psychiatry, University of Rochester Medical Center, Center for the Study and Prevention of Suicide, Rochester, New York

HANNAH WARD, MD
Resident Physician, Department of Internal Medicine, Johns Hopkins Bayview Medical Center, Baltimore, Maryland

TRAVIS P. WELSH, MD
Department of Internal Medicine, UT Southwestern Medical Center, Dallas, Texas

AILING E. YANG, BA
Department of Internal Medicine, UT Southwestern Medical Center, Dallas, Texas

Contents

Vassiliki Pravodelov

Polypharmacy, the use of five or more medications, is common in older adults. It can lead to the use of potentially inappropriate medications and severe adverse outcomes. Deprescribing is an essential step of the thoughtful prescribing process and it can decrease the use of potentially inappropriate medications. Studies have demonstrated that deprescribing is feasible in the clinical setting, especially when it incorporates patient preferences, shared decision making, and an interdisciplinary team. Medication-specific algorithms can facilitate deprescribing in the clinical setting.

Amber Comer, Lyle Fettig, and Alexia M. Torke

Goals of care conversations are important but complex for clinicians caring for older adults. Although clinicians tend to focus on specific medical interventions, these conversations are more successful if they begin with gaining a shared understanding of the medical conditions and possible outcomes, followed by discussion of values and goals. Although training in the medical setting is incomplete, there are many published and online resources that can help clinicians gain these valuable skills.

Mariana R. Gonzalez, Rachel K. Miller, and Alyson R. Michener

Geriatric assessment is a comprehensive, multifaceted, and interdisciplinary evaluation of medical, socioeconomic, environmental, and functional concerns unique to older adults; it can be focused or broadened according to the needs of the patient and the concerns of clinical providers. Herein, the authors present a high-yield framework that can be used to assess older adult patients across a variety of settings.

Colleen M. Casey, Jamie Caulley, and Elizabeth A. Phelan

A large body of research has addressed the assessment and management of fall risk among community-dwelling older adults. Persons with dementia are at higher risk for falls and fall-related injuries, yet less is known about effective strategies for reducing falls and injuries among those with dementia. Falls and dementia are regularly considered to be discrete conditions and are often managed separately. Increasing evidence shows that these conditions frequently co-occur, and one may precede the other. This article explores the relationship between falls and dementia, including the importance of rehabilitation strategies for reducing fall risk in these individuals.

Clinicians should use a systematic approach to evaluating patients presenting with a concern for cognitive impairment. This approach includes interviewing a knowledgeable informant and performing a thorough mental status examination in order to determine the presence of functional impairments and the domains of cognition that are impaired. The results of this interview and examination determine the next steps of the diagnostic work-up. The pattern of cognitive impairment shapes the differential diagnosis. Treatment should address symptoms, and environmental, psychological, and behavioral interventions are essential.

The prevalence of urinary incontinence and other lower urinary tract symptoms increases with older age. These symptoms are more noticeable in men after the seventh decade of life and in women after menopause. Constipation and fecal incontinence are major causes of symptoms in elderly patients and can significantly impair quality of life. This article summarizes the current literature regarding the occurrence and implications of lower urinary tract and bowel symptoms in the geriatric population.

Older adults experience greater emotional well-being in late life. However, older adults may be vulnerable to certain physiologic risk factors, including less physiologic resilience to prolonged stress. Depression and anxiety can be difficult to diagnose in late life owing to differences in self-reported symptoms from younger adults and unclear distinctions between normative and non-normative emotional experiences. We discuss age differences in the presentations of depression and anxiety, and normative and non-normative late life developmental trajectories around bereavement and grief, social isolation and loneliness, and thoughts of death and suicide. We provide recommendations for clinicians for assessing and diagnosing older adults.

Persistent pain in older adults is a widely prevalent and disabling condition that is the manifestation of multiple contributing physical, mental, social, and age-related factors. To effectively treat pain, the clinician must assess and address contributing factors using a comprehensive approach that includes pharmacologic and nonpharmacologic therapies within the context of a strong therapeutic relationship among the patient, caregivers, and a multidisciplinary team. This article reviews the current understanding of persistent pain in older adults and suggests a general approach to its assessment and management, followed by specific considerations for musculoskeletal pain conditions commonly seen in older adults.

capacity each change over time. Transparent decision making and harm reduction help balance risk and safety. When a patient lacks decisional capacity, an option that considers the patient's preferences and shows respect for the person is favored. Vulnerable patients making choices that are high risk, and patients for whom others are making such choices, may require state intervention.

Foreword

Knowledge, Wisdom, and the Practice of Geriatrics

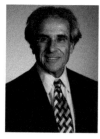

Jack Ende, MD, MACP
Consulting Editor

I wish I knew who actually said, "Knowledge is knowing which way to look when crossing a one-way street; wisdom is looking both ways, nonetheless." I have used that quote so many times, especially on rounds.

An 86-year-old patient is admitted for the third time in 6 months with an exacerbation of congestive heart failure (CHF) manifest by fluid overload. Knowledge of management of CHF directs us to diurese him while monitoring renal function and other parameters. But wisdom moves us to ask, why is he experiencing still another episode of fluid overload? Does he have the medications he requires? Is he taking them? Is he following a salt-restricted diet? The list goes on. Moreover, our inquiry might include more integrative questions, such as, does he and his family understand the natural history of CHF? Should we be focused more on home care, and achieving goals that are both possible and valued by our patient.

No group of physicians appreciates the importance of wisdom, in addition to knowledge, more than do expert geriatricians. They know the most up-to-date, evidence-based guidelines and use them to direct care. But geriatricians also understand that, in addition to guidelines, nothing is more important than personalized care, adjusted to the patient's age, sex, comorbidities, socioeconomic determinants, and, most importantly, the patient's personal goals. That takes wisdom.

Where does wisdom come from? From experience, of course, and also from knowledge of the most recent medical advances and guidelines. Expert geriatricians, however, charged as they are with care of complex, elderly patients with multiple comorbidities and complex living situations, appreciate as much or even more than other subspecialists that high-quality care requires wisdom grounded in knowledge.

So I commend us all to spend time with this issue of *Medical Clinics of North America* "Geriatrics for Internists." It includes up-to-date articles on pharmacology in the elderly, fall prevention, cognitive impairment, bladder and bowel symptoms, chronic

Med Clin N Am 104 (2020) xv–xvi
https://doi.org/10.1016/j.mcna.2020.06.012
0025-7125/20/© 2020 Published by Elsevier Inc.

pain, osteoporosis, and perioperative assessment in the elderly. It also includes articles providing thoughtful advice on identifying goals of care, geriatric assessment, managing sadness and worry in the elderly, symptom management, and challenges related to safety and independence. Our guest editor, Danelle Cayea, has assembled an outstanding group of expert authors. They have reviewed the most recent knowledge and point us in the direction of wisdom. We may not all restrict our practice to geriatrics, but we can provide our elderly patients with the best possible care.

Jack Ende, MD, MACP
Department of Medicine
Perelman School of Medicine
of the University of Pennsylvania
5033 West Gates Pavilion
3400 Spruce Street
Philadelphia, PA 19104, USA

E-mail address:
jack.ende@pennmedicine.upenn.edu

Preface

Caring for Older Adults

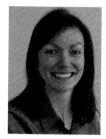

Danelle Cayea, MD, MS
Editor

The planning for this issue of *Medical Clinics of North America* started in 2019, long before "coronavirus," "shelter at home," and "social distancing" became part of our everyday discourse. It feels like a long time since we have been able to routinely see our patients in clinic and meet in person with interdisciplinary teams. Many of the topics covered in this issue are necessarily "high touch" practices. It is unclear when we will be able to partake in some of these practices regularly and consistently again. However, as some older adults have difficulty accessing digital health care, experience increased isolation and loneliness, and face the prospect of hospitalization or intubation if they become ill from the SARS-COV2 virus, it is more imperative than ever that we have a workforce with the skills and knowledge to provide excellent care to older adults. It is yet to be determined what impact delaying care or receiving telehealth care only during the pandemic will have on the health and well-being of older adults, who have the highest rates of chronic health conditions of any age group.

At all times, clinicians must be able to anticipate problems their older patients may be having, screen for them, and effectively diagnose and manage them. In recent times, clinicians must be even more astute in this regard. Take for example an 84-year-old woman with hypertension and type 2 diabetes. She lives alone and has several very close friends she typically sees regularly. She drives and manages her finances easily. Her blood pressure is previously well controlled, and through diet she has maintained her HbA1c in goal range. Since the coronavirus pandemic started, she has been terrified of contracting the virus and has been shopping only every few weeks. This has led to her consuming more carbohydrates and nonperishable foods, with higher salt content. Because she cannot go to the senior center to exercise, she has been spending much of her time sitting and reading. She finds herself aware of some back pain almost daily and is feeling increasingly lonely as she has been sheltering in place. She is having trouble falling asleep at night. She's heard about rationing of ventilators in other countries and isn't sure how she feels about that or whether she

Med Clin N Am 104 (2020) xvii–xviii
https://doi.org/10.1016/j.mcna.2020.06.011
0025-7125/20/© 2020 Published by Elsevier Inc.

should go on one if she became ill. She contacts your office to discuss these concerns but does not think she will be able to figure out the video platform for a telehealth visit. This patient is not an isolated example, and she deserves a team of clinicians who can take a holistic approach to her health and well-being and communicate effectively around these issues.

This issue highlights some of metaskills important to the care of older adults, including an approach to prescribing and deprescribing, identifying and discussing goals of care, and assessing safety and independence. It also includes guidance on the evaluation and management of several common symptoms and diseases seen in older adults, including pain, sadness and worry, falls, urinary and bowel symptoms, osteoporosis, cognitive impairment, and perioperative management.

I am incredibly grateful to the authors for writing such thoughtful and holistic articles during such a professionally and personally challenging time and to the journal for continuing to highlight the importance of providing excellent care to older adults.

Danelle Cayea, MD, MS
Department of Medicine
Johns Hopkins University School of Medicine
4940 Eastern Avenue
Suite 220
Baltimore, MD 21224, USA

E-mail address:
dcayea1@jhmi.edu

Thoughtful Prescribing and Deprescribing

Vassiliki Pravodelov, MD[a,b],*

KEYWORDS

- Polypharmacy • Older adults • Deprescribing
- Potentially inappropriate medications • Shared decision making

KEY POINTS

- Potentially inappropriate medications and polypharmacy have been associated with adverse events in the older adult population.
- Deprescribing is an important element of the thoughtful prescribing process and can help decrease inappropriate polypharmacy.
- Shared decision making and consideration of patient goals are essential for successful deprescribing.
- Algorithms and clinical decision tools are available to assist providers with identifying potentially inappropriate medications and applying the deprescribing process.

OVERVIEW

In this article, we (1) discuss polypharmacy and deprescribing of potentially inappropriate medications (PIMs) in the older adult population; (2) explore the benefits, risks, barriers, and enablers of deprescribing; and (3) review and apply the deprescribing process to a patient case.

INTRODUCTION TO OUR CASE

An 81-year-old woman presents to the clinic for a geriatric assessment. Her medical problems include Parkinson disease complicated by mild dysphagia, knee osteoarthritis complicated by falls, hypertension, and type 2 diabetes mellitus. The patient's main concern is fatigue and difficulty managing a long list of medications. She reports difficulty swallowing multiple pills at the same time, especially "the really large pills." The patient notes that her goal is to improve her current quality of life and functionality

[a] Section of Geriatrics, Department of Medicine, Boston University School of Medicine, 72 East Concord Street, Robinson 2, Boston, MA 02118, USA; [b] Boston Medical Center, One Boston Medical Center Place, Boston, MA 02118, USA
* Section of Geriatrics, Department of Medicine, Boston University School of Medicine, 72 East Concord Street, Robinson 2, Boston, MA 02118.
E-mail address: vpravode@bu.edu

Med Clin N Am 104 (2020) 751–765
https://doi.org/10.1016/j.mcna.2020.06.001
0025-7125/20/© 2020 Elsevier Inc. All rights reserved.

by managing her parkinsonian symptoms as much as possible. She does not want any invasive interventions. On review of the record, the patient's hemoglobin A_{1c} was 5.2% a few weeks before the visit. Her blood pressure is 130/74. The patient has brought in all her medications. She is taking acetaminophen and naproxen for knee osteoarthritis, carbidopa-levodopa for Parkinson disease, losartan for hypertension, metformin for diabetes mellitus, pantoprazole, baby aspirin, simvastatin, and a calcium/vitamin D daily supplement. The patient notes difficulty swallowing metformin, simvastatin, and her calcium/vitamin D supplement because of the size of the tablets. She asks, "Do I need all these medications?"

POLYPHARMACY

Polypharmacy is commonly defined as taking five or more regularly prescribed medications.[1] Studies suggest that polypharmacy is common in older adults.[2,3] This is likely multifactorial. Older adults can have many chronic conditions. Clinical practice guidelines for individual conditions often lead to polypharmacy, which can initially seem rational but may be problematic in older adults with multiple comorbidities; especially because this population is often excluded from trials used to develop clinical practice guidelines.[4] Prescribing cascades (prescribing a medication to manage a side effect of another medication) may also lead to problematic polypharmacy.[5,6]

POTENTIALLY INAPPROPRIATE MEDICATIONS

With a vast number of medications prescribed in the older adult population, the use of PIM is common.[7,8] Potentially inappropriate prescribing may include overprescribing, misprescribing, or underprescribing.[9] As patients age, their physical and functional condition may change, as do their goals of treatment or what matters to them most. Therefore, a medication that had been appropriately prescribed in the past may become inappropriate later in life because of its risks outweighing any potential benefits for the particular patient.

Polypharmacy and the use of PIM is harmful in older adults with studies showing its association with decreased quality of life and increased adverse drug reactions, falls, hospitalizations, and mortality.[10] Budnitz and colleagues[11] identified the medications and medication classes accounting for the most emergency department visits for adverse drug events among older adults in the United States. Warfarin, insulin, oral antiplatelet agents, and oral antihyperglycemics topped the list.

As part of the Choosing Wisely campaign, the American Geriatrics Society recommended conducting a medication reconciliation before prescribing a medication to identify polypharmacy and PIMs.[12]

Several tools have been published to assist with the identification of PIMs. In the United States, the Beers Criteria was first published in 1991 and it includes medications that can cause adverse effects in the geriatric population and therefore, should be avoided or used with caution. The most recent update, the 2019 AGS Beers Criteria for Potentially Inappropriate Medication Use in Older Adults, includes a comprehensive list of medications and drug classes whose risks may outweigh their benefits in older adults in general and in conjunction with specific comorbidities.[13]

In addition, the STOPP (Screening Tool of Older Person's Prescriptions) and START (Screening Tool to Alert Doctors to Right Treatment) screening tools can help providers identify PIMs.[14–16] In 2015, experts from seven European countries published the EU(7)-PIM list containing PIMs for older adults along with dose adjustments and therapeutic alternatives.[17]

Table 1 lists commonly prescribed medication classes that may be inappropriate because of their potential for harm in older adults.[13,14,17]

WHAT IS DEPRESCRIBING?

In response to the prevalence of polypharmacy and inappropriate prescribing, deprescribing was suggested as a method to minimize harm.[31] Deprescribing is defined as the positive patient-centered process of stopping or reducing the dose of medications that are considered inappropriate for a particular patient because their risks outweigh their potential benefits, they are unnecessary, or they are ineffective.[32] The deprescribing process is supervised and directed by a health care professional through shared decision making and its goal is to manage polypharmacy and reduce harm according to patient priorities.[31,32]

Common reasons to consider deprescribing medications in the geriatric population are listed in **Table 2**.

DEPRESCRIBING: BENEFITS AND RISKS

Deprescribing, as a response to polypharmacy and inappropriate prescribing, is believed to reduce harm associated with PIMs. A systematic review by Page and

Table 1 Common medication classes that may be inappropriate in older adults because of their potential for harm	
Medication Class	**Potential Risks**
Proton pump inhibitors[13,14,17–19]	Osteoporotic fractures *Clostridium difficile* infection Kidney injury
Benzodiazepines[13,14,17,20,21]	Confusion Falls

Antihyperglycemics[13,14,17,22–24]	Depending on pharmacologic class
	  Hypoglycemia
	  Pancreatitis (GLP-1 receptor antagonists, DPP-4 inhibitors)
	  Worsening heart failure symptoms (DPP-4 inhibitors)
	  Genitourinary infections (SGLT2)

Cholinesterase inhibitors[14,25–27]	Gastrointestinal symptoms Bradycardia Confusion
Antipsychotics[13,14,17,28]	Increased risk of stroke, cognitive decline, and mortality in patients with dementia
Nonsteroidal anti-inflammatory drugs[13,14,17,29]	Gastrointestinal bleeding Kidney injury Hypertension
Anticholinergics[13,14,17,30]	Confusion Dry mouth Constipation and urinary retention
Nonbenzodiazepine hypnotics[13–15,17,30]	Confusion Falls

Data from Refs.[13,14,17–30]

Table 2
When to consider deprescribing in older adults

Reasons for Deprescribing	Clinical Examples
Medication risks outweigh potential benefits	β-Blocker used in a patient with orthostatic hypotension and multiple falls. Trimethoprim-sulfamethoxazole prescribed for a patient with chronic kidney disease who is already taking an angiotensin-converting enzyme inhibitor.
Medication may be inappropriate (PIM)	Zolpidem used for insomnia in a patient with falls. Sulfonylurea used in a patient with aberrant feeding pattern and frequent hypoglycemic episodes.
Medication is not necessary	Chronic proton pump inhibitor used in an asymptomatic patient. The medication was started 2 y ago for acid reflux, which has since resolved. Daily multivitamin in an asymptomatic patient without malnutrition.
Medication is ineffective	Cholinesterase inhibitors used for years for a patient with end-stage dementia without providing an observed additional benefit.
Medication is burdensome and difficult to adhere to	Medications that must be administered multiple times daily (eg, hydralazine, carvedilol, labetalol) when other alternatives exist to decrease burden and improve adherence.
Medication does not align with patient wishes	Multiple medication classes used per guideline recommendations for one condition (eg, heart failure) but patient's primary goal is to minimize polypharmacy and pill burden.
Medication time-to-benefit inconsistent with patient prognosis	Preventive medications used in patients on hospice care (eg, statin, aspirin).
Medication may be contributing to an adverse drug effect	Symptomatic bradycardia in a patient with dementia who was started on donepezil.

Data from Refs.[13,18,31–33]

colleagues[34] determined that, among nonrandomized studies, deprescribing was found to decrease mortality. Among randomized studies, deprescribing did not have a significant effect on mortality.[34]

Studies have shown that deprescribing may be beneficial for patients with limited life expectancy. For example, in Kutner and colleagues[35] patients whose life expectancy was less than 12 months had no mortality difference at 60 days if statin was deprescribed. Furthermore, patients who stopped statin had a significantly better quality of life. Statin deprescribing for older adults who are not at their end of life remains controversial.[36,37]

Risks of deprescribing include the possibility of rebound or withdrawal symptoms. A Cochrane review of deprescribing antipsychotics in patients with dementia showed that stopping an antipsychotic may be feasible and may have a minor important effect on behavioral symptoms and cognitive function. The authors, however, note that two

---

Box 1

Patient-related barriers to deprescribing

- Fear of adverse drug withdrawal effects
- Fear of changing the "status quo"
- Disagreement with deprescribing reasoning
- Negative "influences" to deprescribe medication (eg, previously told they should take the medication "for the rest of their life," influence from family/caregivers/friends)
- Absence of a deprescribing process

Data from Refs.[41–44]

---

of the included studies, who only included patients who had responded to antipsychotic treatment, suggested an increased risk of rebound symptoms after discontinuation of antipsychotics.[38]

Overuse and misuse of proton pump inhibitors (PPI) have been described in the literature, especially with rising concerns regarding possible adverse effects with their long-term use.[18] Studies suggest that, despite the risk of rebound symptoms, deprescribing PPIs is feasible, especially if medication tapering is used.[39,40]

BARRIERS TO DEPRESCRIBING

Surveys among patients and providers have described several barriers to deprescribing.[41,42] Some of the most important barriers identified in the literature are summarized in **Boxes 1** and **2**.

Box 2

Provider-related barriers to deprescribing

- Assumption that patient/caregiver is not interested in deprescribing
- Fear of adverse drug withdrawal effects
- Fear of changing the "status quo"
- Difficulty with medication reconciliation (patient receiving medications from multiple providers, multiple pharmacies, multiple institutions)
- Reassigning responsibility to another provider
- Pressure from clinical practice guidelines to prescribe
- Lack of skills in identifying and managing polypharmacy, PIM, and deprescribing
- Lack of time: clinic visits are too short and deprescribing may not be the most pressing issue on the agenda
- Lack of organizational support: deprescribing requires effort and close monitoring
- Concern that effective alternatives are not available
- Fear of consequences in quality measures
- Ambiguity regarding feasibility of deprescribing
- Unclear medication indication

Data from Refs.[41,42,45]

ENABLERS FOR DEPRESCRIBING

Studies suggest that patient-centered interventions for deprescribing are more effective than non-patient-centered interventions.[46] Patients are interested in reducing the number of medications they take if their provider thought it would be possible.[43] Therefore, engaging the patient and/or caregiver in the deprescribing process is crucial for its success. Jansen and colleagues[47] described a four-step deprescribing process for older adults focused on shared decision making: (1) creating deprescribing awareness, (2) discussing options, (3) exploring patient preferences, and (4) making the decision.

Including a multidisciplinary team with clinical pharmacists and/or nursing staff for close monitoring can help with the logistical constraints faced by primary care clinicians. Interdisciplinary teams, such as The Geriatric Patient-Aligned Care Team (GeriPACT) in the Veteran Affairs system, have shown promise in augmenting the deprescribing process in older adults.[48]

THE PROCESS OF DEPRESCRIBING

Deprescribing is an essential element of the thoughtful prescribing process. When a medication is prescribed, its effectiveness, indication, potential benefits and harms, and alignment with the patient's preferences should be reassessed at regular intervals to ensure its appropriateness.[49]

The literature includes multiple different approaches to deprescribing. Deprescribing interventions can take place in various settings (outpatient, long-term care, inpatient)[50,51] and target different patient populations (older adults, patients at the end of life, patients with cognitive impairment, cancer, human immunodeficiency virus, chronic kidney disease).[21,46,52–60]

Most deprescribing processes in the literature emphasize the importance of patient/caregiver involvement (or "buy-in") in the deprescribing process. Reeve and colleagues[31] summarized the importance of "consumer involvement" in the process. Ouellet and colleagues[58] described a rational prescribing and deprescribing process based on "what matters" most to older patients while weighing the risks and benefits of medications. This is achieved through shared decision making. In a recent article, Green and colleagues[57] described helpful language that can facilitate conversations between clinicians and patients/caregivers to improve appropriate prescribing.

Essential steps of the deprescribing process based on the available literature were collected and visually summarized in **Fig. 1**.[19,20,22,28,31–33,46,47,61]

PRACTICAL PRESCRIBING AND DEPRESCRIBING RESOURCES IN THE CLINIC

Multiple resources are available to assist clinicians with deprescribing. Canada, Australia, and several European countries have developed extensive online resources, many of which are free to use[62–65]. The Canadian Deprescribing Network[66] is well-established and its website includes a plethora of practical clinician-oriented algorithms, patient handouts, and educational videos (https://deprescribingnetwork.ca). In the United States, the US Deprescribing Research Network (USDeN) was launched in November 2019. The USDeN is funded by the US National Institute of Aging and it aims to help promote deprescribing research in order to improve appropriate medication use among older adults.[67] Its website (https://deprescribingresearch.org/) contains links to useful online deprescribing resources for practicing clinicians, investigators, as well as patients.

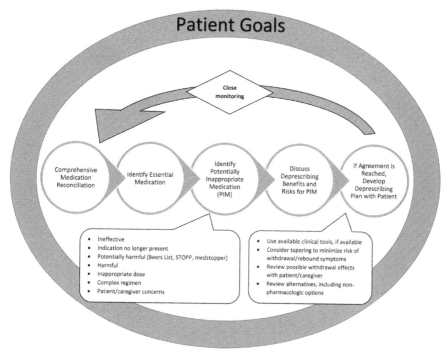

Fig. 1. Deprescribing process.

APPLYING THE DEPRESCRIBING PROCESS TO OUR CASE

Our patient has multiple chronic medical conditions and a long medication list. Next we apply the steps of the deprescribing process as shown in **Fig. 1**.

Detailed medication reconciliation is done using the "brown bag" method.[68] We identify potentially essential medications. We also find that the patient is experiencing polypharmacy and PIMs: her list contains medications that may be contributing to her presenting symptoms, medications that may no longer be indicated, medications without an associated diagnosis, and medications whose benefits may no longer outweigh their risks.

On discussion with the patient, we discover that she has concerns about how her current medications may be affecting her everyday life and how they may be contributing to some of her symptoms (dysphagia, fatigue, falls). She would like to simplify her medication list if her clinical providers think it would be possible.

We then take a closer look at her medication list and we identify areas to further clarify with the patient. These are listed in **Table 3**.

We work with the patient to prioritize her concerns and develop a deprescribing plan. Based on what matters most to the patient and our previous medication-related discussion, we agree on the following deprescribing plan:

- It is unclear what is causing her fatigue but hypoglycemia may be contributing. In 2019, the American Diabetes Association suggested that A_{1c} goals for older adults are less stringent (<7.5%–8.5% depending on comorbidities, cognitive function, and functional status).[24] Her A_{1c} (5.2%) is well below her goal based on her age and comorbidities. Besides, the patient has difficulty swallowing the medication because of its size. Therefore, as a first step, it is reasonable to stop metformin. The patient readily agrees to stop metformin but is worried about

Table 3
Polypharmacy and PIM concerns for the patient

Medication	Concerns	Patient Clarification	PIM?
Acetaminophen	Appropriate dose? Effective?	The patient says she takes this as needed, 325 mg at a time. She does not use it more than twice daily. She is not sure if it is effective.	
Naproxen	Appropriate dose? Any adverse events?	The patient takes this when the knee pain is worse than usual, about twice a month. She takes it twice daily during flare-ups. She finds it worrisome that it could make her hypertension worse.	
Carbidopa-levodopa	Appropriate dose? Effective? Monitored by a neurologist?	She takes the medication as prescribed by her neurologist, 4 times daily. She notices improvement in stiffness after taking the medication. She last saw her neurologist 3 months ago and has an upcoming appointment next month.	
Losartan	Any adverse events, such as dizziness?	It is hard to tell whether she has any dizziness after taking this because she takes it with most of her other medications. She has been taking this medication for more than 10 y now.	
Metformin	Any adverse events, such as dizziness, fatigue, dyspepsia? Burdensome?	She is uncertain if she has any dizziness after taking this because she takes it with most of her other medications. She has a hard time swallowing the pill because of its large size. The patient is wondering if there is a smaller pill formulation for her to try.	

Medication	Questions	Details	
Pantoprazole	Indication for use? Appropriate administration?	She is not sure why she is taking this. The patient reports she had acid reflux in the past but has not had any symptoms in years. She has never been diagnosed with esophagitis, Barrett esophagus, or peptic ulcer disease. She takes the medication before breakfast.	◀●
Aspirin	Indication for use? Any adverse effects, such as acid reflux or gastrointestinal bleed?	The patient is not sure why she is taking this. She was told by her doctor years ago that she has to take it "for life" to protect her heart. She has never had a heart attack or a stroke. She had acid reflux symptoms in the past, now resolved. She has not noticed any blood in her stool.	◀●
Simvastatin	Indication for use? Burdensome? Any adverse effects, such as muscle aches?	She is not sure why she is taking this. She does note difficulty swallowing the medication because of its size. She has not noticed any persistent muscle aches.	◀●
Calcium/vitamin D	Indication for use? Burdensome?	She started taking this years ago because she heard that calcium and vitamin D can help keep her bones strong. She obtains it over the counter. The patient says she had a test for osteoporosis a year ago and it was normal. Calcium and vitamin D levels are within normal levels.	◀●

her diabetes control. We discuss lifestyle modifications (nonconcentrated sweets diet, exercise) and plan to monitor closely.[22]

- The patient's use of naproxen is problematic. Chronic nonsteroidal anti-inflammatory drug (NSAID) use has been associated with various adverse events including kidney injury, hypertension, and gastrointestinal ulcers.[69,70] NSAIDs have a Boxed Warning regarding serious cardiovascular thrombotic events, such as myocardial infarction and stroke.[71] We discuss the risks and benefits of use with the patient. She does not think that the medication's benefits outweigh its potential risks and we remove the medication from her list. However, she is concerned about pain management during flare-ups. We review alternatives, including appropriate use and dosing of acetaminophen, nonpharmacologic interventions (eg, physical therapy), and topical analgesics. The patient is open to trying diclofenac gel as needed during flare-ups.
- The patient has a significant pill burden and some medications lack an indication: pantoprazole, aspirin, simvastatin, and calcium/vitamin D supplementation. Given that we are already implementing two high-priority changes with metformin and naproxen, we review our options with the patient. She feels comfortable stopping the calcium/vitamin D supplementation because she finds the tablet difficult to swallow because of its size. We recommend foods rich in calcium that she can include in her diet.

By the end of our visit, naproxen, metformin, and calcium/vitamin D have been stopped, whereas diclofenac gel has been added for pain control. The medication changes are communicated with her pharmacy.

A week after our visit, the clinic nurse makes an outreach telephone call to the patient to review medications and address any concerns. A month later, the patient returns for a comprehensive medication review follow-up with our clinical pharmacist. She has not had any adverse withdrawal events and her quality of life has improved since our last visit: her medication list is down to six pills and one topical gel and her fatigue has improved. The clinical pharmacist continues the discussion regarding risks and benefits of aspirin, simvastatin, and pantoprazole use with the patient. The patient is not ready to stop another medication at this time but she is open to continuing medication appropriateness discussions at subsequent visits.

SUMMARY

Thoughtful prescribing and deprescribing are aspects of the same continuum. Recognizing opportunities for intervention and engaging the patient and caregiver in the interdisciplinary process may prove rewarding for patients and providers. Although several tools are available to enable thoughtful prescribing and deprescribing, more research is needed to fill in the gaps and provide further practical guidance for front-line clinicians.

CLINICS CARE POINTS

- PIMs and polypharmacy are associated with adverse events in the older adult population.
- Clinical tools are available to identify PIMs.
- Deprescribing is an important element of the thoughtful prescribing process.
- Shared decision making and awareness of patient preferences are essential for successful deprescribing.
- Multidisciplinary teams can enhance the deprescribing process.

- Deprescribing algorithms and decision aids are available for several medication classes including PPIs, antihyperglycemics, antipsychotics, cholinesterase inhibitors, and benzodiazepines.

DISCLOSURE

The author has nothing to disclose.

REFERENCES

1. Gnjidic D, Hilmer SN, Blyth FM, et al. Polypharmacy cutoff and outcomes: five or more medicines were used to identify community-dwelling older men at risk of different adverse outcomes. J Clin Epidemiol 2012;65(9):989–95.
2. Qato DM, Wilder J, Schumm LP, et al. Changes in prescription and over-the-counter medication and dietary supplement use among older adults in the United States, 2005 vs 2011. JAMA Intern Med 2016;176(4):473–82.
3. Kantor ED, Rehm CD, Haas JS, et al. Trends in prescription drug use among adults in the United States from 1999-2012. JAMA 2015;314(17):1818–31.
4. Molokhia M, Majeed A. Current and future perspectives on the management of polypharmacy. BMC Fam Pract 2017;18. https://doi.org/10.1186/s12875-017-0642-0.
5. Rochon PA, Gurwitz JH. Optimising drug treatment for elderly people: the prescribing cascade. BMJ 1997;315(7115):1096–9.
6. Rochon PA, Gurwitz JH. The prescribing cascade revisited. Lancet 2017;389(10081):1778–80.
7. Renom-Guiteras A, Thürmann PA, Miralles R, et al. Potentially inappropriate medication among people with dementia in eight European countries. Age Ageing 2018;47(1):68–74.
8. Secora A, Alexander GC, Ballew SH, et al. Kidney function, polypharmacy, and potentially inappropriate medication use in a community-based cohort of older adults. Drugs Aging 2018;35(8):735–50.
9. O'Connor MN, Gallagher P, O'Mahony D. Inappropriate prescribing. Drugs Aging 2012;29(6):437–52.
10. Wastesson JW, Morin L, Tan ECK, et al. An update on the clinical consequences of polypharmacy in older adults: a narrative review. Expert Opin Drug Saf 2018;17(12):1185–96.
11. Budnitz DS, Lovegrove MC, Shehab N, et al. Emergency hospitalizations for adverse drug events in older Americans. N Engl J Med 2011. https://doi.org/10.1056/NEJMsa1103053.
12. American Geriatrics Society | Choosing Wisely. Available at: https://www.choosingwisely.org/societies/american-geriatrics-society/. Accessed January 30, 2020.
13. By the 2019 American Geriatrics Society Beers Criteria® Update Expert Panel. American Geriatrics Society 2019 updated AGS beers criteria® for potentially inappropriate medication use in older adults. J Am Geriatr Soc 2019;67(4):674–94.
14. Gallagher P, Ryan C, Byrne S, et al. STOPP (screening tool of older person's prescriptions) and START (screening tool to alert doctors to right treatment). Consensus validation. Int J Clin Pharmacol Ther 2008;46(2):72–83.
15. Hamilton H, Gallagher P, Ryan C, et al. Potentially inappropriate medications defined by STOPP criteria and the risk of adverse drug events in older hospitalized patients. Arch Intern Med 2011;171(11):1013–9.

16. Hill-Taylor B, Sketris I, Hayden J, et al. Application of the STOPP/START criteria: a systematic review of the prevalence of potentially inappropriate prescribing in older adults, and evidence of clinical, humanistic and economic impact. J Clin Pharm Ther 2013;38(5):360–72.

17. Renom-Guiteras A, Meyer G, Thürmann PA. The EU(7)-PIM list: a list of potentially inappropriate medications for older people consented by experts from seven European countries. Eur J Clin Pharmacol 2015;71(7):861–75.

18. Al-Aly Z, Maddukuri G, Xie Y. Proton pump inhibitors and the kidney: implications of current evidence for clinical practice and when and how to deprescribe. Am J Kidney Dis 2019. https://doi.org/10.1053/j.ajkd.2019.07.012.

19. Farrell B, Pottie K, Thompson W, et al. Deprescribing proton pump inhibitors: evidence-based clinical practice guideline. Can Fam Physician 2017;63(5): 354–64.

20. Pottie K, Thompson W, Davies S, et al. Deprescribing benzodiazepine receptor agonists: evidence-based clinical practice guideline. Can Fam Physician 2018; 64(5):339–51.

21. Reeve E, Ong M, Wu A, et al. A systematic review of interventions to deprescribe benzodiazepines and other hypnotics among older people. Eur J Clin Pharmacol 2017;73(8):927–35.

22. Farrell B, Black C, Thompson W, et al. Deprescribing antihyperglycemic agents in older persons: evidence-based clinical practice guideline. Can Fam Physician 2017;63(11):832–43.

23. Gonzalez-Perez A, Schlienger RG, Rodríguez LAG. Acute pancreatitis in association with type 2 diabetes and antidiabetic drugs. Diabetes Care 2010;33(12): 2580–5.

24. Association AD. 12. Older adults: standards of medical care in diabetes—2019. Diabetes Care 2019;42(Supplement 1):S139–47.

25. Campbell NL, Perkins AJ, Gao S, et al. Adherence and tolerability of Alzheimer's disease medications: a pragmatic randomized trial. J Am Geriatr Soc 2017;65(7): 1497–504.

26. Hernandez RK, Farwell W, Cantor MD, et al. Cholinesterase inhibitors and incidence of bradycardia in patients with dementia in the Veterans Affairs New England healthcare system. J Am Geriatr Soc 2009;57(11):1997–2003.

27. Reeve E, Farrell B, Thompson W, et al. Deprescribing cholinesterase inhibitors and memantine in dementia: guideline summary. Med J Aust 2019;210(4):174–9.

28. Bjerre LM, Farrell B, Hogel M, et al. Deprescribing antipsychotics for behavioural and psychological symptoms of dementia and insomnia: evidence-based clinical practice guideline. Can Fam Physician 2018;64(1):17–27.

29. Marsico F, Paolillo S, Filardi PP. NSAIDs and cardiovascular risk. J Cardiovasc Med (Hagerstown) 2017;18:e40–3. Suppl 1: Special Issue on The State of the Art for the Practicing Cardiologist: The 2016 Conoscere E Curare Il Cuore (CCC) Proceedings from the CLI Foundation.

30. Ailabouni N, Mangin D, Nishtala PS. Deprescribing anticholinergic and sedative medicines: protocol for a feasibility trial (DEFEAT-polypharmacy) in residential aged care facilities. BMJ Open 2017;7(4):e013800.

31. Reeve E, Thompson W, Farrell B. Deprescribing: a narrative review of the evidence and practical recommendations for recognizing opportunities and taking action. Eur J Intern Med 2017;38:3–11.

32. Scott IA, Hilmer SN, Reeve E, et al. Reducing inappropriate polypharmacy: the process of deprescribing. JAMA Intern Med 2015;175(5):827.

33. Hardy JE, Hilmer SN. Deprescribing in the last year of life. J Pharm Pract Res 2011;41(2):146–51.
34. Page AT, Clifford RM, Potter K, et al. The feasibility and effect of deprescribing in older adults on mortality and health: a systematic review and meta-analysis. Br J Clin Pharmacol 2016;82(3):583–623.
35. Kutner JS, Blatchford PJ, Taylor DH, et al. Safety and benefit of discontinuing statin therapy in the setting of advanced, life-limiting illness: a randomized clinical trial. JAMA Intern Med 2015;175(5):691–700.
36. Han BH, Sutin D, Williamson JD, et al. Effect of statin treatment vs usual care on primary cardiovascular prevention among older adults: the ALLHAT-LLT randomized clinical trial. JAMA Intern Med 2017;177(7):955–65.
37. Singh S, Zieman S, Go AS, et al. Statins for primary prevention in older adults-moving toward evidence-based decision-making. J Am Geriatr Soc 2018; 66(11):2188–96.
38. Leeuwen EV, Petrovic M, Driel ML van, et al. Withdrawal versus continuation of long-term antipsychotic drug use for behavioural and psychological symptoms in older people with dementia. Cochrane Database Syst Rev 2018;(3). https://doi.org/10.1002/14651858.CD007726.pub3.
39. Kim J, Blackett JW, Jodorkovsky D. Strategies for effective discontinuation of proton pump inhibitors. Curr Gastroenterol Rep 2018;20(6):27.
40. Haastrup P, Paulsen MS, Begtrup LM, et al. Strategies for discontinuation of proton pump inhibitors: a systematic review. Fam Pract 2014;31(6):625–30.
41. Reeve E, To J, Hendrix I, et al. Patient barriers to and enablers of deprescribing: a systematic review. Drugs Aging 2013;30(10):793–807.
42. Paque K, Vander Stichele R, Elseviers M, et al. Barriers and enablers to deprescribing in people with a life-limiting disease: a systematic review. Palliat Med 2019;33(1):37–48.
43. Reeve E, Wolff JL, Skehan M, et al. Assessment of attitudes toward deprescribing in older Medicare beneficiaries in the United States. JAMA Intern Med 2018; 178(12):1673.
44. Linsky A, Meterko M, Bokhour BG, et al. Deprescribing in the context of multiple providers: understanding patient preferences. Am J Manag Care 2019;25(4): 192–8.
45. Linsky A, Meterko M, Stolzmann K, et al. Supporting medication discontinuation: provider preferences for interventions to facilitate deprescribing. BMC Health Serv Res 2017;17. https://doi.org/10.1186/s12913-017-2391-0.
46. Todd A, Jansen J, Colvin J, et al. The deprescribing rainbow: a conceptual framework highlighting the importance of patient context when stopping medication in older people. BMC Geriatr 2018;18. https://doi.org/10.1186/s12877-018-0978-x.
47. Jansen J, Naganathan V, Carter SM, et al. Too much medicine in older people? Deprescribing through shared decision making. BMJ 2016;i2893. https://doi.org/10.1136/bmj.i2893.
48. Potentially inappropriate medications in older adults: deprescribing with a clinical pharmacist. Available at: https://www.ncbi.nlm.nih.gov/pubmed/30300947. Accessed January 30, 2020.
49. Endsley S. Deprescribing unnecessary medications: a four-part process. Fam Pract Manag 2018;25(3):28–32.
50. Ailabouni N, Mangin D, Nishtala PS. DEFEAT-polypharmacy: deprescribing anticholinergic and sedative medicines feasibility trial in residential aged care facilities. Int J Clin Pharm 2019;41(1):167–78.

51. Vasilevskis EE, Shah AS, Hollingsworth EK, et al. A patient-centered deprescribing intervention for hospitalized older patients with polypharmacy: rationale and design of the Shed-MEDS randomized controlled trial. BMC Health Serv Res 2019;19(1):165.
52. Martin P, Tamblyn R, Ahmed S, et al. An educational intervention to reduce the use of potentially inappropriate medications among older adults (EMPOWER study): protocol for a cluster randomized trial. Trials 2013;14:80.
53. McNicholl IR, Gandhi M, Hare CB, et al. A pharmacist-led program to evaluate and reduce polypharmacy and potentially inappropriate prescribing in older HIV-positive patients. Pharmacotherapy 2017;37(12):1498–506.
54. Martin P, Tamblyn R, Benedetti A, et al. Effect of a pharmacist-led educational intervention on inappropriate medication prescriptions in older adults: the D-PRESCRIBE randomized clinical trial. JAMA 2018;320(18):1889–98.
55. Whitman A, DeGregory K, Morris A, et al. Pharmacist-led medication assessment and deprescribing intervention for older adults with cancer and polypharmacy: a pilot study. Support Care Cancer 2018;26(12):4105–13.
56. Harrison SL, Cations M, Jessop T, et al. Approaches to deprescribing psychotropic medications for changed behaviours in long-term care residents living with dementia. Drugs Aging 2019;36(2):125–36.
57. Green AR, Wolff JL, Echavarria DM, et al. How clinicians discuss medications during primary care encounters among older adults with cognitive impairment. J Gen Intern Med 2020;35(1):237–46.
58. Ouellet GM, Ouellet JA, Tinetti ME. Principle of rational prescribing and deprescribing in older adults with multiple chronic conditions. Ther Adv Drug Saf 2018; 9(11):639–52.
59. McIntyre C, McQuillan R, Bell C, et al. Targeted deprescribing in an outpatient hemodialysis unit: a quality improvement study to decrease polypharmacy. Am J Kidney Dis 2017;70(5):611–8.
60. Potter EL, Lew TE, Sooriyakumaran M, et al. Evaluation of pharmacist-led physician-supported inpatient deprescribing model in older patients admitted to an acute general medical unit. Australas J Ageing 2019;38(3):206–10.
61. Stopping medicines in older people: the flip side of the prescribing equation - bpacnz. Available at: https://bpac.org.nz/2018/stopping.aspx. Accessed January 30, 2020.
62. Deprescribing.org - Optimizing Medication Use. Available at: https://deprescribing.org/. Accessed January 30, 2020.
63. MedStopper. Available at: http://medstopper.com/. Accessed January 30, 2020.
64. Deprescribing resources - Primary Health Tasmania. Available at: https://www.primaryhealthtas.com.au/resources/deprescribing-resources/. Accessed January 30, 2020.
65. Polypharmacy Guidance - Medicines Review. Available at: http://www.polypharmacy.scot.nhs.uk/polypharmacy-guidance-medicines-review/. Accessed January 30, 2020.
66. Do I still need this medication? Is deprescribing for you? Do I still need this medication? Is deprescribing for you? Available at: https://www.deprescribingnetwork.ca. Accessed June 16, 2020.
67. Home - US Deprescribing Research Network. Available at: https://deprescribingresearch.org/. Accessed January 30, 2020.
68. Caskie GIL, Willis SL, Warner Schaie K, et al. Congruence of medication information from a brown bag data collection and pharmacy records: findings from the Seattle longitudinal study. Exp Aging Res 2006;32(1):79–103.

69. Gunter BR, Butler KA, Wallace RL, et al. Non-steroidal anti-inflammatory drug-induced cardiovascular adverse events: a meta-analysis. J Clin Pharm Ther 2017;42(1):27–38.
70. Harirforoosh S, Asghar W, Jamali F. Adverse effects of nonsteroidal antiinflammatory drugs: an update of gastrointestinal, cardiovascular and renal complications. J Pharm 2013;16(5):821–47.
71. Research C for DE and. FDA Drug Safety Communication: FDA strengthens warning that non-aspirin nonsteroidal anti-inflammatory drugs (NSAIDs) can cause heart attacks or strokes. FDA. 2019. Available at: http://www.fda.gov/drugs/drug-safety-and-availability/fda-drug-safety-communication-fda-strengthens-warning-non-aspirin-nonsteroidal-anti-inflammatory. Accessed January 30, 2020.

Identifying Goals of Care

Amber Comer, JD, PhD[a], Lyle Fettig, MD[b], Alexia M. Torke, MD, MS[c],*

KEYWORDS

- Goals of care • Geriatrics • Palliative care • Ethics

KEY POINTS

- Decision making for older adults is complicated by increased prevalence of serious illness, complexity caused by comorbidities, and decisions that are sensitive to the individual preference of patients.
- Goals of care conversations should explore values, goals, and treatment preferences.
- Needed clinician training can be attained through structured programs. Many resources are publicly available.

INTRODUCTION

As a person ages or faces serious illness, decisions about medical care become more challenging. When cure of a disease is not possible, treatments become focused on other goals such as symptom amelioration or extending life. Additionally, both the underlying disease and the treatments may cause suffering to the patient. Finally, as patients age, the outcomes of medical interventions are more uncertain because of comorbidities or frailty. Because individuals are more likely to differ in their preferences for or against treatment in these circumstances, decisions are often referred to as preference sensitive.[1] Preference-sensitive decisions vary based on the individual values, goals and circumstances of the patient.

The term goals of care is commonly used to refer to the entire process of making medical decisions, but it really has several components, including values, goals, and treatment preferences (**Fig. 1**). It can involve making decisions for the future, often referred to as advance care planning, or making decisions about medical treatment in the present. Such conversations can occur in the hospital, nursing home, and outpatient setting. In this article, the authors will describe a framework for addressing goals

[a] School of Health and Human Sciences, Indiana University, 1050 Wishard Boulevard, RG 3034, Indianapolis, IN 46202, USA; [b] Division of General Medicine and Geriatrics, Palliative Care, Indiana University School of Medicine, Eskenazi Health, 640 Eskenazi Avenue, Indianapolis, IN 46202, USA; [c] Division of General Medicine and Geriatrics, Indiana University School of Medicine, Indiana University Center for Aging Research, Regenstrief Institute, Incorporated, 1101 West 10th Street, Indianapolis, IN 46202, USA
* Corresponding author.
E-mail address: atorke@iu.edu
Twitter: @AlexiaMTorke (A.M.T.)

Med Clin N Am 104 (2020) 767–775
https://doi.org/10.1016/j.mcna.2020.06.002
medical.theclinics.com

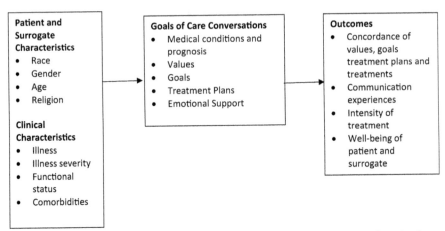

Fig. 1. Model of the patient and surrogate factors, process, and outcomes of goals of care conversations.

of care, review literature on communication about goals, and review important outcomes such as medical treatments received and patient or family psychological outcomes.

As patients age, their ability to make their own decisions is more likely to be impaired because of dementia, and delirium is a common cause of diminished capacity during acute illness. Therefore surrogate decision makers, usually close family members, often are involved in the decision-making process. Goals of care conversations for older adults may be held with patients, surrogates, or both, but can consider the same core components. Surrogates are generally asked to rely on the patient's previously stated preferences, when known. When specific preferences are unknown, surrogates are asked to consider how the patients' goals and values should inform treatment decisions, a process called substituted judgment.[2] Although surrogate decision making introduces additional ethical and emotional considerations, the approach involves many of the same concepts and skills as goals of care conversations with patients.

Goals of care conversations require physicians to effectively communicate complex information about a medical diagnosis and its prognosis to the patient and family, elicit information about patient preferences, provide support and make shared decisions, and ensure treatments and outcomes are aligned with patient and family preferences. The struggle for clinicians to have goals of care conversations is particularly important for geriatric providers, as the need to communicate prognosis and set goals of care to alleviate suffering is both time sensitive and common. These conversations are sometimes conducted by palliative care specialists who are experts in goals of care conversations, but often these conversations are conducted by the patient's primary physician or hospitalists. These communication challenges arise at high rates during end-of-life care, when decisions are more preference sensitive. Effective goals of care conversations usually explore values and preferences prior to considering specific treatment interventions.

TERMINOLOGY
Values

Values are broad concepts that guide one's actions, and may include the value of life, family connections, or living according to religious or cultural beliefs and traditions.

Balancing quality of life against length of life is a trade-off that must be considered for some highly burdensome treatments. In exploring values, clinicians may ask, "What is most important to you?" or "What gives your life meaning?" For some patients and families, values are closely related to religious or spiritual traditions, and chaplains may be especially valuable in elucidating or clarifying them. The Interprofessional Spiritual Care Educational Curriculum (ISPEC) is a curriculum developed to train nonchaplains how to address spiritual concerns when they arise and to promote collaboration between chaplains and various clinicians, including physicians, to provide comprehensive spiritual care to patients.[3]

Physicians also have deeply held values such as promoting health and reducing suffering.[4] In the vast majority of patient care, patient and physician values are concordant. However, when outcomes are uncertain or the burden of treatment increases, there may be ethical conflicts between clinician and patient values. Resources such as ethics or palliative care consultation may be valuable and will be described.

Patient-Defined Goals

Studies that ask patients to describe their own goals for medical care have identified categories such as cure, being comfortable, or remaining at home.[5] Goals may be broad or specific, but most importantly are defined by the patient or his or her surrogate. Exploring goals in advance of treatment decisions will help clinicians understand patient motivations for or against particular treatments.

Discussions should focus on the patient's or surrogates' personal goals or the overarching goals of treatment, such as preserving life or focusing on comfort. Examples include being able to recover enough to engage in meaningful conversation, being comfortable, or living to a specific event. Using open-ended questions to ask patients about their own goals can help foster communication about specific treatments. Affirming patient goals can be a positive way to connect and build trust. Sometimes patient's stated goals may be impossible or uncertain. Physicians can probe further, by asking about additional hopes. By taking the approach of "hoping for the best but preparing for the worst," clinicians can partner with patients and families while also assisting in making realistic plans for medical treatment.[6]

Treatment Preferences

In counseling patients, an important role of the physician is to explore how a particular treatment will help the patient attain his or her goals and is concordant with his or her values.[7]

Ethical challenges arise when patients select inconsistent plans of treatment. Incoherent plans have the potential to cause patient suffering while not achieving goals.

These include categories of treatment and specific decisions about individual interventions A 3-part framework is helpful in research and clinical care to describe treatment preferences[8–10] The 3 general categories are: treatment focused on keeping the patient comfortable, usually by providing pain and symptom management; an intermediate plan of care involving hospitalization, intravenous (IV) medications or monitoring; and full, life-sustaining treatments including ventilators, dialysis, and major surgery. Research on treatment preferences has found that decision aids and videos may help improve patient understanding of goals of care and may lead to more documented goals of care conversations.[8,9] When properly informed, patients may be more likely to receive comfort-focused interventions.[11]

The most specific level of treatment decision making involves a particular intervention such as a surgery or medication. These should generally be considered in light of the broader categories of values, goals, and general treatment preferences as well as medical evidence and expert opinion about the value of a particular treatment. In the primary care setting, older adults are at risk for polypharmacy, ordering of duplicative or unnecessary testing, and referrals for potentially unwanted evaluations. The American Geriatrics Society has joined the Choosing Wisely campaign, making a series of recommendations about specific treatments, with the goals of reducing burdensome polypharmacy and the ordering of screening tests that are unlikely to benefit older adults.[12]

THE CLINICAL CONTEXT

There is ample evidence that culture, race, and religion play a role in goals of care and in treatments patients receive (see **Fig. 1**). There are some general trends of which clinicians should be aware. On average, African American patients and more highly religious patients and families tend to prefer more life-sustaining treatments in serious illness.[13,14] However, many patients from these groups do want and receive high quality comfort care as illness progresses.[15,16] Asking questions about the patient's individual priorities and the individual values of the patient is essential.

The goals of care also depend on the clinical situation and prognosis. Knowing the likely outcomes of the patient's condition and the range of options is essential to the decision-making process. Among geriatric patients, clinical features such as frailty and functional status vary widely from patient to patient. Comorbidities also complicate estimates of prognosis for older adults.[17] These factors may contribute to estimates of patient outcomes being inconsistent across different providers. In some cases, prognostic calculators can help a clinician estimate prognosis in order to guide goals of care discussions.[18,19] Many of these calculators are easily available online.[20] An essential responsibility of the physician is to evaluate these factors prior to conversations with the patient so that the patient can be educated about his or her condition, and realistic goals can be set. Studies have found that patients and caregivers desire different amounts of information, with patients often wanting less information, and caregivers wanting more. Clinicians should be attuned to the patient's desire for information and ability to understand. Teach-back or Ask-Tell-Ask is a useful approach to confirm understanding.[21]

TREATMENT PLANS

After a goals of care conversation, decisions need to be communicated and translated into medical treatments. Appropriately documenting the decisions made and the reasons for the decisions can be important to future decision making. The decision may lead to proceeding with a surgery, a hospital admission, or other major intervention. Treatment planning also involves deciding ahead of time about emergent interventions such as code status or intubation. Such decisions can be documented by do not resuscitate (DNR) orders in the hospital or do not hospitalize orders in the nursing home setting. An important tool for documenting these types of treatment preferences is the Physicians Orders for Life Sustaining Treatment (POLST) paradigm and form.[10] POLST has the advantage of transferring across settings such as the nursing home or community. Legally valid POLST forms are available in nearly all US states, although the names of the form and the treatment choices vary. POLST forms include preferences for 3 categories of medical interventions (comfort-focused treatments, intermediate or selective treatments, and life-sustaining or full interventions). Patients also indicate preferences for cardiopulmonary resuscitation. Some states include preferences for antibiotics or artificial nutrition. Unlike advance directives, POLST forms are medical orders that must be signed by a physician (or nurse practitioner or physician assistant in some states). There are frameworks that guide the conversations about POLST forms such as Respecting Choices Advanced Steps, in which a trained facilitator guides a patient through a conversation to identify values, goals, and treatment preferences.[22]

OUTCOMES OF GOALS OF CARE CONVERSATIONS

High-quality decision making involves considering specific treatment preferences in the context of values, goals and treatment preferences. Defining a good outcome requires exploring an individual patient's perceptions about quality of life, because individuals often have different viewpoints on whether death or survival with disability is the better outcome. Therefore an important outcome of this process is that treatments are concordant with patient values and preferences.[5,23,24] Additionally, it is then important that concordance is achieved between preferences and the treatments that the patient actually receives.[25]

CLINICIAN TRAINING AND RESOURCES

A recent survey of primary care physicians and medical subspecialists who regularly see older adults revealed that 68% of physicians report no training related to talking with patients about goals and wishes at the end of life.[26] This was despite nearly universal consensus among survey participants that it is important to have end-of-life conversations. During medical education, communication training often occurs passively through observation of more senior physicians and trainee trial and error. Because faculty may not be well versed in best communication practices or teaching principles, bedside teaching may be subject to the hidden curriculum with the risk of transmitting bad habits. When seeing patients who are under stress from serious illness and face complex value-sensitive decisions that are mired by uncertainty, well-trained faculty physicians can teach communication through role modeling and coaching. There is a high need for communications skills training to ensure that providers are matching treatments to seriously ill patient goals and values.[27]

As goals of care conversations frequently occur during clinical worsening, patients often experience difficult emotions during conversations. Clinicians should expect strong emotions when delivering bad news or talking about goals of care. Patients and families can be supported by actions that convey empathy, including acknowledging patient emotion, allowing some silence when the patient expresses emotion, and statements that suggest partnering and nonabandonment.[28] By conveying empathy, physicians can ensure that conversations remain focused on achievable patient-oriented quality-of-life goals and values, even when other goals may not be achievable. When the patient raises unachievable goals, physician empathy can be used to provide grief support and resolve conflict.[28,29] There is also evidence that even though spiritual and religious supports are important to patients and benefit them, physicians often ignore these issues when patients and families raise them.[30]

Another useful framework, REMAP (Reframe, Expect Emotion, Map the future, Align with patient values, Plan treatment) framework was developed to provide physicians with a step-by-step process for goals of care conversations when there is a change in condition.[31] This guide may be especially helpful to clinicians who are learning to conduct these conversations but also to experienced clinicians to ensure that all important components of the conversation are addressed. This framework, along with the NURSE (Naming, Understanding, Respecting, Supporting, Exploring) mnemonic for responding to emotion, has been used extensively for simulation practice and coaching. The use of simulated patients encourages physicians to reflect on the individual communication skills important for each step in the process of goals of care conversations. Rapid-cycle deliberate practice and debriefing that promote learner experimentation with new strategies allow learners to compare various strategies.[32,33] Many institutions have incorporated simulation into medical education curricula, and opportunities exist for continuing education for practicing physicians. This teaching format has been demonstrated to increase physician use of high-yield skills, including jargon-free discussion of the patient's condition, verbal empathy, and open exploration of concerns.[34]

In older adults, high-stakes decision making about treatment options often requires comparison between a potentially invasive or burdensome intervention (eg, surgery) with unclear outcomes and an alternative path of supportive care. Decision aids may be valuable in communicating with patients about options. The Best Case/Worst Case (BC/WC) tool provides patients with a side-by-side comparison of options, with a best case, worst case, and most likely case narrative description of the anticipated course with each option.[35] With a brief 2-hour workshop, a group of surgeons was able to implement this tool with reasonable fidelity, with most surgeons reporting use of the tool after 6 months. Patients report that the graphic aid facilitates deliberation and allows comparison between treatment options, establishing expectations about a range of outcomes.

Early consideration of goals, values, and treatment preferences in the outpatient setting can prevent older adults from undergoing unwanted interventions and help them discuss their priorities with surrogate decision makers. The Serious Illness Conversation Guide (SICG) was developed as an aid to discussions in the clinic, typically outside the setting of an acute illness. A training workshop is available to implement this guide, which relies on question prompts that ask patients to reflect on their goals and values. Common electronic medical record systems in the United States have integrated this guide to promote documentation, and a particular strength of the SICG is consideration of system integration. There are several other published and online resources that address goal development,[7,36] reducing burdensome treatments and tests unlikely to benefit older adults (Choosing Wisely) and supporting spiritual and religious needs of patients and families (**Table 1**).

SPECIALTY CONSULTATION IN GOALS OF CARE

Goals of care conversations have the potential to raise difficult ethical issues and can lead to conflict between families, patients and clinicians, and even among clinicians. Clinicians may experience moral distress, the feeling that they know the right thing to do but are constrained from carrying it out. Discordance among values, goals, and treatments can be an important source of moral distress and ethical conflict. In such cases, palliative care consultations and ethics consultations can help to readdress decision making. Additionally, when emotional or religious concerns are prominent, social workers and chaplains can play a role in providing support and navigating the decision-making process.

DISCUSSION AND SUMMARY

Goals of care conversations are important but complex for clinicians caring for older adults. Although clinicians tend to focus on specific medical interventions, these conversations are more successful if they begin with gaining a shared understanding of the medical conditions and possible outcomes, followed by discussion of values and goals. Although training in the medical setting is incomplete, there are many published and online resources that can help clinicians gain these valuable skills.

Table 1
Published and online resources for clinicians having goals of care conversations with geriatric patients.

Name	Access	Description
Respecting Choices	Access to materials is through agreement with Respecting Choices www.respectingchoices.org	Provides training for structured facilitation of advance care planning
Vitaltalk	www.vitaltalk.org	Training for physicians and others leading goals of care conversations
VALUE framework	Publication[29]	Communication strategies to improve decision making
Serious Illness Care	https://www.ariadnelabs.org/areas-of-work/serious-illness-care/	A program and guide to improve communication, includes the serious illness communication guide
Best case/Worst case	Publication[35]	Communication tool for side-by-side comparison of options, and narrative description of the anticipated course with each option
Patient Priorities Care	Publication[7]	Deliberate evaluation of patient values and the development of SMART goals (specific, measurable, actionable, reliable, and time bound) to drive medical decision-making

Data from Refs.[7,29,35]

CLINICS CARE POINTS

Goals of care conversations should address the clinical situation, patient values, and patient goals before discussing specific medical treatments. Clinicians should be prepared to respond to emotion with empathy and to acknowledge and support religious and spiritual needs.

Providing patents and families the opportunity to talk about their concerns will increase satisfaction with the process. Ethics and palliative care consultation can help resolve challenges with decision making about goals of care and related treatments. Social work and chaplaincy are integral to providing ongoing support to patients.

DISCLOSURE

Dr. Torke was supported by a Patient Midcareer Investigator Award in Patient Oriented Research (K24AG053794) from the National Institute on Aging.

REFERENCES

1. O'Connor AM, Wennberg JE, Legare F, et al. Toward the 'tipping point': decision aids and informed patient choice. Health Aff (Millwood) 2007;26:716–25.

2. Buchanan AE, Brock DW. Deciding for others: the ethics of surrogate decision making. Cambridge: Cambridge University Press; 1989.

3. Puchalski C, Jafari N, Buller H, et al. Interprofessional spiritual care education curriculum: a milestone toward the provision of spiritual care. J Palliat Med 2020;23(6):777–84.

4. Kaldjian LC. Teaching practical wisdom in medicine through clinical judgement, goals of care, and ethical reasoning. J Med Ethics 2010;36:558–62.

5. Kaldjian LC, Curtis AE, Shinkunas LA, et al. Goals of care toward the end of life: a structured literature review. Am J Hosp Palliat Care 2008;25:501–11.

6. Back AL, Arnold RM, Quill TE. Hope for the best, and prepare for the worst. Ann Intern Med 2003;138:439–43.

7. Tinetti ME, Naik AD, Dodson JA. Moving from disease-centered to patient goals–directed care for patients with multiple chronic conditions: patient value-based care. JAMA Cardiol 2016;1:9–10.

8. Volandes AE, Brandeis GH, Davis AD, et al. A randomized controlled trial of a goals-of-care video for elderly patients admitted to skilled nursing facilities. J Palliat Med 2012;15:805–11.

9. Mitchell SL, Shaffer ML, Cohen S, et al. An advance care planning video decision support tool for nursing home residents with advanced dementia: a cluster randomized clinical trial. JAMA Intern Med 2018;178:961–9.

10. Physician Orders for Life-Sustaining Treatment Paradigm. Available at: http://www.polst.org/. Accessed December 13, 2013.

11. Hanson LC, Zimmerman S, Song MK, et al. Effect of the goals of care intervention for advanced dementia: a randomized clinical trial. JAMA Intern Med 2017;177:24–31.

12. Available at: https://www.choosingwisely.org/societies/american-geriatrics-society/. Accessed February 27, 2020.

13. Phelps AC, Maciejewski PK, Nilsson M, et al. Religious coping and use of intensive life-prolonging care near death in patients with advanced cancer. JAMA 2009;301:1140–7.

14. Hong M, Yi E, Johnson KJ, et al. Facilitators and barriers for advance care planning among ethnic and racial minorities in the U.S.: a systematic review of the current literature. J Immigr Minor Health 2018;20:1277–87.

15. Born W, Greiner KA, Sylvia E, et al. Knowledge, attitudes, and beliefs about end-of-life care among inner-city African Americans and Latinos. J Palliat Med 2004;7:247–56.

16. Torke AM, Garas NS, Sexson W, et al. Medical care at the end of life: views of African American patients in an urban hospital. J Palliat Med 2005;8:593–602.

17. Boyd CM, Darer J, Boult C, et al. Clinical practice guidelines and quality of care for older patients with multiple comorbid diseases: implications for pay for performance. JAMA 2005;294:716–24.

18. Lee SJ, Lindquist K, Segal MR, et al. Development and validation of a prognostic index for 4-year mortality in older adults. JAMA 2006;295:801–8.

19. Gagne JJ, Glynn RJ, Avorn J, et al. A combined comorbidity score predicted mortality in elderly patients better than existing scores. J Clin Epidemiol 2011;64:749–59.

20. ePrognosis. Available at: www.ePrognosis.ucsf.edu. Accessed March 17, 2017.

21. Teach Ba/kc. Available at: http://www.teachbacktraining.org/to-learn-more. Accessed February 25, 2020.

22. Respecting choices: person centered care. Available at: https://respectingchoices.org/. Accessed January 23, 2019.

23. Johnson SB, Butow PN, Kerridge I, et al. How well do current measures assess the impact of advance care planning on concordance between patient preferences for end-of-life care and the care received: a methodological review. J Pain Symptom Manage 2018;55:480–95.

24. Cohen SM, Volandes AE, Shaffer ML, et al. Concordance between proxy level of care preference and advance directives among nursing home residents with advanced dementia: a cluster randomized clinical trial. J Pain Symptom Manage 2018;57(1):37–46.e1.

25. Carnahan JL, Unroe KT, Torke AM. Hospital readmission penalties: coming soon to a nursing home near you! J Am Geriatr Soc 2016;64(3):614–8.

26. Fulmer T, Escobedo MB, A.B., et al. Physicians' views on advance care planning and end-of-lifecare conversations. J Am Geriatr Soc 2018;66:1201–5.

27. Back AL, Fromme EK, Meier DE. Training clinicians with communication skills needed to match medical treatments to patient values. J Am Geriatr Soc 2019; 67:S435–41.

28. Vitaltalk. Available at: http://www.vitaltalk.org/. Accessed July 13, 2020.

29. Curtis JR, White DB. Practical guidance for evidence-based ICU family conferences. Chest 2008;134:835–43.

30. Ernecoff NC, Curlin FA, Buddadhumaruk P, et al. Health care professionals' responses to religious or spiritual statements by surrogate decision makers during goals-of-care discussions. JAMA Intern Med 2015;175:1662–9.

31. Childers JW, Back AL, Tulsky JA, et al. REMAP: a framework for goals of care conversations. J Oncol Pract 2017;13:e844–7.

32. Fryer-Edwards K, Wilkins MD, Baernstein A, et al. Bringing ethics education to the clinical years: ward ethics sessions at the University of Washington. Acad Med 2006;81:626–31.

33. Chancey RJMS, Esther M, Lemke DS. Learners' experiences during rapid cycle deliberate practice simulations a qualitative analysis. Simul Healthc 2019;14: 18–28.

34. Back AL, Arnold RM, Baile WF, et al. Efficacy of communication skills training for giving bad news and discussing transitions to palliative care. Arch Intern Med 2007;167:453–60.

35. Kruser J, Nabozny MJ, Steffens NM, et al. "Best case/worst case:" qualitative evaluation of a novel communication tool for difficult in-the-moment surgical decisions. J Am Geriatr Soc 2015;63:1805–11.

36. Bradley EH, Bogardus ST, Tinetti ME, et al. Goal-setting in clinical medicine. Soc Sci Med 1999;49:267–78.

Overview of High Yield Geriatrics Assessment for Clinic and Hospital

Mariana R. Gonzalez, MD, MPH, Rachel K. Miller, MD, MsEd*,
Alyson R. Michener, MD

KEYWORDS

- Geriatric assessment • Geriatrics • Functional status • Cognition
- Geriatric syndromes • Polypharmacy

KEY POINTS

- Geriatric assessment is critical for all providers, in the hospital, in the clinic, or in the home care setting, to consider in caring for older adults.
- Geriatric assessment should focus on careful evaluation of older patients' cognition and physical function and should include an assessment for common geriatric syndromes.
- As part of a comprehensive geriatric assessment, providers should provide a careful assessment of patients' medications and be able to identify medications that may put older patients at risk for adverse events.
- Geriatric assessment should be tailored to patient values and goals and take into consideration multimorbidity and life expectancy.

INTRODUCTION

Older adults face unique social and health challenges, and, as the population of the United States continues to age, it is critical that practitioners are able to develop and use a framework for assessing older adults. Geriatric assessment refers to the comprehensive, multifaceted, and interdisciplinary evaluation of medical, socioeconomic, environmental, and functional concerns that are unique to older adults. Data from several investigations demonstrate that comprehensive geriatric assessment, especially for patients in the inpatient setting, offer significant benefit for older adults despite higher cost; patients who underwent geriatric assessment were more likely to survive hospitalization and remain in their own home after discharge.[1] Although providers may perceive it to be challenging to care for older adults, geriatric assessment can provide a helpful framework by which to evaluate multimorbidity, ultimately

Division of Geriatrics, University of Pennsylvania, 3615 Chestnut Street, Philadelphia, PA 19104, USA
* Corresponding author.
E-mail address: Rachel.Miller@uphs.upenn.edu

Med Clin N Am 104 (2020) 777–789
https://doi.org/10.1016/j.mcna.2020.06.005
0025-7125/20/Published by Elsevier Inc.

medical.theclinics.com

allowing providers to more easily and safely manage medical complaints, uncover social or economic issues that may impact medical care, and provide high-value care according to patients' goals and priorities.[2]

A geriatric assessment can take place in a variety of settings, including in the home, in the clinic, in the hospital, or in the rehabilitation setting, and may require a brief, focused examination or a more extensive, broader review within a larger number of domains, depending on the needs of the patient and the concerns of the clinician. A geriatric assessment should be a team-based effort and include collaboration among team members in pharmacy, nursing, social work, and rehabilitation (including occupational, physical, and speech therapy). The Medicare Annual Wellness Visit provides an opportunity to screen for concerns requiring further exploration in many of the domains covered in a comprehensive geriatric assessment.

COMPONENTS OF A COMPREHENSIVE GERIATRIC ASSESSMENT
Function, Cognition, and Assessment for Geriatric Syndromes

In assessing older adults, priority should be given to screening for common geriatric syndromes, constellations of clinical concerns that may cause significant morbidity for older adult patients. **Table 1** summarizes brief assessment tools that can be used in the evaluation of older patients.

Table 1 Common geriatric syndromes and commonly used evaluation tools	
Functional assessment	ADLs/IADLs Katz Index of Independence in Activities of Daily Living Lawton Instrumental Activities of Daily Living Scale
Cognitive impairment Dementia	Mini-Cog (screening) Montreal Cognitive Assessment (MoCA) Mini Mental State Examination (MMSE) Saint Louis University Mental Status Exam (SLUMS)
Delirium	CAM CAM-ICU
Depression	PHQ-2 Geriatric Depression Scale (GDS)
Falls	Timed get-up-and-go
Urinary incontinence	Michigan Incontinence Symptom Index (M-ISI)
Nutritional assessment	Mini Nutritional Assessment—Short Form (MNA-SF) Short Nutritional Assessment Questionnaire (SNAQ)

Functional Assessment

Functional status refers to patients' ability to perform the tasks necessary to meet their basic daily needs. Chronic disease often results in functional limitations and disability. Because a significant portion of older adults lives with chronic disease, it is important for the clinician to perform an assessment of an older adult's function. Clinicians may use this information to identify remediable conditions, the types of assistance needed, and potential interventions to allow the older adult to maintain independence.[3] In addition, functional status correlates with quality of life and is a predictor of longevity.[4]

Functional abilities have been classified as basic activities of daily living (ADLs) and instrumental activities of daily living (IADLs) (**Table 2**). ADLs include tasks that are

Table 2
Functional abilities: activities of daily living and instrumental activities of daily living

Activities of Daily Living	Instrumental Activities of Daily Living
Bathing	Using the telephone
Dressing	Preparing meals
Transferring	Laundry
Toileting	Housework/cleaning
Grooming	Shopping
Feeding	Transportation
	Managing medications
	Finances

necessary for maintaining basic self-care on a daily basis. IADLs include tasks necessary to maintain independence in a community.

A comprehensive geriatric assessment should include evaluation of an older adult's ability to perform the tasks listed in **Table 2**. The Katz Index of Independence in Activities of Daily Living and the Lawton Instrumental Activities of Daily Living Scale are tools that have been developed to assist the clinician in measuring functional status.[5]

Deficits in ADLs and IADLs occur when there is disconnect between patients' capabilities and their environmental demands. Inability to perform any of these tasks independently should prompt further assessment and rehabilitation, which often requires consultation from interdisciplinary team members, including physical and occupational therapy.[6] The clinician should also consider what, if any, supports are currently in place to help patients accomplish such tasks. Such supports may include delegation to a caregiver, environmental modifications, or even nursing home placement.

Gait, Balance, and Falls

Falls are a common cause of injury in older adults and, therefore, risk factors should be considered part of a functional assessment for all geriatric patients. In performing this part of the geriatric assessment, clinicians should ask their patients about a history of falls in the last year, fear of falling, or whether they perceive any balance or gait problems. A positive answer to any of these questions should prompt further investigation to identify potential risk factors.[7]

A variety of both extrinsic and intrinsic factors may put an older adult at risk of falling, but assessment of transfers, gait, and balance has the advantage of being easily observable in a variety of clinical settings. Much can be gleaned from observing an older patient rise from a seated position and ambulate several feet. Rising from a seated position requires core and proximal muscle strength. Some patients may experience postural hypotension, which can be evaluated with orthostatic vital signs. Features of an older adult's gait, including balance, speed, arm swing, and turns, may also provide useful information and should be closely observed.

The "timed get-up-and-go" is a validated tool whereby the older adult must stand from a seated position, ambulate 10 feet, turn around, walk back, and return to a seated position while being timed by the observer. A time of greater than 12 seconds has been linked to a greater risk of falls.[8] In addition, gait speed less than 0.8 m per second has also been shown to be predictive of falls, frailty, and mortality in older adults.[9]

Cognition and Mental Health

Changes in memory and cognitive function commonly go underrecognized in older patients. These changes can have significant impact on older adults' ability to manage medical comorbidities, perform necessary ADL, and successfully remain independent and active in their community.

In assessing cognitive impairment, providers should ask patients about any concerns about their memory function. Because many patients may not notice or report memory concerns, and there can be some social stigma surrounding memory loss, it may be important to obtain collateral information from patients' caretakers or family members about any memory impairments. The Mini-Cog, which includes a 3-word recall and a clock draw test, is a brief screening examination for cognitive impairment and may be performed rapidly in the office or the inpatient setting in order to identify patients who may require further workup of cognitive concerns.[10]

Dementia

For patients who express concerns about their memory and also demonstrate impairments in their daily function, providers should consider further evaluation for a cognitive disorder. First, providers should take care to rule out the possibility of underlying medical or "reversible" causes that may result in cognitive changes, such as electrolyte abnormalities or untreated medical conditions (ie, infection, arrhythmia, or thyroid disorders), and patients should be screened for signs and symptoms of delirium. Acute mood disorders, such as depression or anxiety, should be addressed, because these may contribute to cognitive decline. Patients with memory concerns should also undergo assessment of hearing and vision complaints. Evaluation of dementia should include a thorough physical examination, including a full neurologic assessment.

Several cognitive tests evaluate the severity of cognitive impairment and identify the specific cognitive domains affected. The Montreal Cognitive Assessment, the Mini Mental State Examination, and the Saint Louis University Mental Status Examination are short evaluations that are commonly used as first-line testing in patients with reported memory concerns.[11–13]

A patient's clinical situation and description of symptoms should be reviewed in order to guide further assessment and testing needs. Basic evaluation may include complete blood counts, metabolic panel, thyroid-stimulating hormone, vitamin levels, or glucose and hemoglobin A1c level. Providers should consider performing brain imaging (such as noncontrast computed tomographic scan or MRI) if there is a concern for recent fall or injury (ie, to evaluate for an acute process, such as a subdural hematoma), or new or localizing neurologic symptoms (which might suggest acute cerebrovascular accident or Parkinsonism). Any patient with findings concerning for rapidly progressive memory loss may require urgent evaluation for more rare causes of dementia.

Delirium

Delirium is a common occurrence, particularly for older adults in the inpatient (hospital) setting, and has been noted to contribute to increased length of hospital stay as well as higher risk for post–hospital institutionalization (ie, nursing home placement). Commonly, delirium is seen as a postoperative complication in older adults, although it can also be seen in the intensive care unit (ICU), in the emergency room, or in palliative care or hospice setting in patients who are approaching the end of life.

Delirium is defined as an acute, reversible change in attention, awareness, and cognition. It may fluctuate in severity (and is notably separate from any preexisting dementia). It may present with signs of significant agitation or psychomotor overactivity ("hyperactive delirium") or with symptoms like somnolence, sedation, and slow speech and movements ("hypoactive delirium").[14]

Assessment of older adult patients, especially in the hospital setting, should include screening for delirium with the Confusion Assessment Method (CAM) tool; the CAM-ICU tool may be used to assess ICU patients.[15,16] The basic treatment for delirium should focus mostly on minimizing aspects of the physical environment that may contribute to delirium: ensuring appropriate sleep-wake cycle and minimizing disruption of sleep (ie, by limiting overnight interventions, such as vital signs monitoring), encouraging cognitive stimulation by family members or nursing staff, ensuring patients have appropriate assistive devices, such as hearing aids and glasses, and removing medical devices like urinary catheters, intravenous catheters, and telemetry monitors when appropriate. Medical interventions should focus on treating underlying medical issues that may contribute to acute confusion, such as treating infections and ensuring management of constipation or urinary retention, appropriate treatment of and prevention of pain, and avoidance or restriction of medications that may contribute to delirium (such as benzodiazepines, opioids, anticholinergics, antipsychotics, and so forth) (**Box 1**).

Mood

Depression and other related mood disorders may be underidentified and untreated in older adults.[17,18] The US Preventive Services Task Force recommends that all adults, including older adults, receive periodic screening for depression; for most patients, the Patient Health Questionnaire-2(PHQ-2) is a useful, quick, and easy screening test that may be used in older adults.[19,20] The Geriatric Depression Scale (GDS) is a longer, validated tool for depression screening in older adults.[21] Patients who have underlying chronic illnesses, psychosocial stressors, a history of depression or other psychiatric illness, and those who live in long-term care facilities may be at increased risk for developing depression. Providers should monitor these patients carefully for changes in mood. Patients' caregivers, such as family members or care providers (like home health aides or visiting nurses), may also be useful in reporting clinical symptoms of depression.

For patients with mood concerns, it is critical for providers to conduct a thorough social history, including a history of recent or remote alcohol and substance abuse. Providers should be sure to ask about other associated symptoms, such as sleep and appetite. A positive PHQ-2 or GDS assessment, report of a personal history of

---

Box 1
Strategies for management and prevention of delirium in older adults

Treatment of underlying/precipitating medical issues

Removal of unnecessary medical devices (intravenous catheters, urinary catheters, and so forth)

Ensuring appropriate sleep-wake cycle (ie, limiting sleep disruption)

Encourage normalization of daytime routine (out of bed, ambulating if able)

Social stimulation (nursing staff, family, friends, and so forth)

Treat and prevent pain

Discontinue or limit medications that may contribute to delirium

Ensure access to appropriate assistive devices (glasses, hearing aids)

depression or other underlying psychiatric disorder, or the presence of severe psychiatric symptoms should prompt further psychiatric assessment.

Other Geriatric Syndromes

Vision impairment

Visual impairment can be a significant concern for older adults and can play a large role in older patients' ability to successfully age in the community. Patients should be asked about recent changes in their vision or perceived decrease in visual acuity; ophthalmologic history, including use of glasses or bifocal lenses, should be obtained. Routine ophthalmologic assessment and visual acuity testing should be encouraged. Poor vision can contribute to low mood and social isolation and may put patients at risk for harm as a risk factor for falls; patients expressing concern about low vision should be referred for ophthalmologic assessment, and providers should consider formal home safety assessment or modifications for patients with significant visual impairment.

Hearing impairment

Age-related hearing loss is common among older adults and may have significant impact on patients. Poor hearing is known to be a risk factor for dementia and may contribute to social isolation and depression.[22,23] Patients and family members should be asked about hearing concerns, and providers should encourage formal hearing assessment and, if indicated, consideration for hearing assistive devices (such as hearing aids).

Weight loss and nutritional assessment

A geriatric assessment should include a review of the patient's weight and diet. Patients may perform a "dietary recall," which may help the practitioner to understand the frequency and content of meals. If there is a concern for weight loss, providers may perform a review of systems, including constitutional symptoms, such as fevers or night sweats, dental concerns (such as caries and tooth pain), and gastrointestinal symptoms (such as dysphagia, odynophagia, abdominal pain, vomiting, changes in bowel habits), which may guide further assessment. Assessment of potentially contributing medications or medical comorbidities should be performed by clinicians, and providers should consider further assessment by a registered dietitian or nutritionist if there are concerns in regards to dietary intake. For patients who report dental concerns, referral to a dentist may be required, especially in patients who may require adjustment of dentures or other dental devices. Patients should be asked about financial stressors, access to food, and possible food insecurity, and, if necessary, providers should work to identify food resources for patients in need. Providers may perform a brief nutritional assessment or administer a malnutrition screening tool (such as the Mini Nutritional Assessment short-form or Short Nutritional Assessment Questionnaire) to better assess older patients' risk for malnutrition and weight loss.[24,25]

Incontinence

Urinary incontinence is a common geriatric syndrome that can severely impact older patients' quality of life, and urinary incontinence can also represent a significant concern for caregivers of older patients. Patients should be asked about urinary symptoms, such as urinary frequency, urgency, voiding patterns (including daytime and nighttime voiding), and fluid intake; utilization of a urinary incontinence screening tool, such as the Michigan Incontinence Symptom Index, may be useful.[26] Patients concerned about urinary issues should have a thorough medication review, with particular focus placed on use and timing of diuretics, as well as anticholinergic medications, such as antidepressants, antipsychotics, opioids, and benzodiazepines, which may contribute to urinary retention.

Older adults may also experience fecal incontinence, and providers should also ask patients about their usual bowel function, regularity, and ability to maintain control of bowel movements.

Polypharmacy and Medication Review

A careful medication review is an essential part of a geriatric assessment. Polypharmacy, defined as the simultaneous use of multiple medications, increases older patients' risk for medication interactions, adverse side effects, poor adherence, and increased financial burden; polypharmacy may also contribute to increased health care–related costs.[27] Performing a "brown-bag" review, in which the patient brings their medication bottles to each appointment with a provider, can serve as a useful tool to ensure patients are filling and taking their prescriptions appropriately, and may help providers uncover potential safety issues because of old or expired prescriptions, duplicate prescriptions, or other inaccuracies in a patient's medication list.

In addition, older adults may be at increased risk for adverse events for common medications. The Beer's criteria proposes a list of medications that may potentially be inappropriate for use in older adults because of a high risk of side effects or adverse events and can serve as a reference for identifying potentially high-risk medications[28] (**Table 3**). An additional resource for providers is the STOPP-START (Screening Tool of Older Persons' Prescriptions–Screening Tool to Alert to Right Treatment) criteria, which provides an evidence-based review in support of (or against) the use of certain medication classes for specific clinical indications.[29]

It is important to consider other factors that may make medication management challenging for older adults. For example, memory disorders or poor cognitive function may make medication adherence challenging for patients. Poor vision also may present a challenge for patients who may need to visualize pill bottle instructions, for individuals who rely on visual function for dosing of medications (ie, for drawing up insulin in a syringe), or for reading medication instructions. The Medi-Cog is 1 tool that may be used in the ambulatory setting to determine a patient's ability to safely manage their medications.[30]

Additional Components of a Comprehensive Geriatric Assessment

Routine health maintenance

As for all patients, health maintenance should be systematically and routinely reviewed as part of routine care for older adults. One opportunity to do so is during the Medicare Wellness Visit. This annual visit is free to Medicare beneficiaries and provides an opportunity for clinicians to perform a health risk assessment and develop a personalized prevention plan.

Cancer screening can be a difficult topic for clinicians to discuss with their older patients, in part because of challenging conversations that may arise when taking patients' overall health, medical comorbidities, and life expectancy into consideration for cancer screening decisions. The American Board of Internal Medicine's "Choosing Wisely" campaign recommends that providers take into consideration individual patients' life expectancy when considering whether to offer cancer screening, although in practice, both clinicians and patients have described a lack of comfort in navigating these conversations.[31,32] A trusting physician-patient relationship, with clear understanding of the patient's personal and health-related goals and preferences, is critical in making decisions about screening for breast, colorectal, lung, or prostate cancer.[33]

Table 3
2019 Beers criteria–selected medications that may cause harm in older adults

Class of Medication	Potential Harm

Antihistamines, first generation
  Chlorpheniramine
  Diphenhydramine
  Hydroxyzine
  Meclizine
  Promethazine
	Anticholinergic side effects (confusion, dry mouth, constipation)

Antispasmodics
  Dicyclomine
  Scopolamine
	Anticholinergic side effects; uncertain effectiveness

Antipsychotics, first and second generation	Increased risk of stroke; increased mortality in patients with dementia

Benzodiazepines
  Alprazolam
  Clonazepam
  Diazepam
  Lorazepam
	Increased risk of cognitive impairment, delirium, falls, fractures

Benzodiazepine receptor agonist hypnotics
  Eszopiclone
  Zaleplon
  Zolpidem
	Increased risk of delirium, falls, fractures; minimal improvement in sleep latency and duration

Clonidine	Adverse central nervous system effects, bradycardia, orthostasis
Digoxin	Increased risk of toxic effects; avoid using as first-line agent for atrial fibrillation or heart failure
Megestrol	Minimal effect on weight; increased risk of thrombotic events
Metoclopramide	Extrapyramidal effects, including tardive dyskinesia
Muscle relaxants Cyclobenzaprine	Anticholinergic effects; sedation; increased risk of fractures; questionable effectiveness
Nifedipine, immediate release	Hypotension, myocardial ischemia
Nitrofurantoin	Avoid if creatinine clearance <30 due to increased risk of toxicity

Nonsteroidal anti-inflammatory drugs , non-cyclooxygenase-selective
  Diclofenac
  Ibuprofen
  Indomethacin
  Meloxicam
  Naproxen
	Increased risk of gastrointestinal bleeding or peptic ulcer disease; can increase blood pressure and induce kidney injury

Peripheral alpha-1 blockers
  Doxazosin
  Prazosin
  Terazosin
	High risk of orthostasis

Proton-pump inhibitors Omeprazole	Avoid scheduled use >8 wk (unless high-risk patient) due to risk of

(continued on next page)

Table 3 (continued)	
Class of Medication	**Potential Harm**
Pantoprazole Lansoprazole Esomeprazole	*Clostridioides difficile* infection, bone loss, and fractures
Sliding scale insulin without concurrent use of basal insulin	Higher risk of hypoglycemia without improvement in hyperglycemia management
Sulfonylureas, long-acting Glimepiride Glyburide	Higher risk of severe prolonged hypoglycemia
Tricyclic antidepressants Amitriptyline Nortriptyline	Anticholinergic side effects; sedation; orthostatic hypotension

Data from 2019 American Geriatrics Society Beers Criteria Update Expert Panel. American Geriatrics Society 2019 Updated AGS Beers Criteria for Potentially Inappropriate Medication Use in Older Adults. J Am Geriatr Soc. 2019 Apr; 67 (4): 674-694.

Clinicians should ensure that older patients are receiving other appropriate preventive health interventions, in particular, vaccinations for influenza, pneumococcal pneumonia, herpes zoster (shingles), and pertussis (whooping cough); other routine vaccinations should be considered according to an individual patient's needs and medical comorbidities.[34]

Providers should be sure to discuss other routine health maintenance concerns that may often be overlooked in older adults, such as sexual health (and concerns about sexual function), and tobacco, alcohol, and other substance use.

Physical activity

The US Department of Health Guidelines recommend 150 minutes of moderate- to high-intensity physical activity weekly for most older and younger adults as part of a healthy lifestyle. For older adults, the guideline further recommends multicomponent physical activity, including balance, strength training, and aerobic exercise.[35] Physical activity has many health benefits, which together can reduce disease and disability while improving quality of life, including decreased risk of early death, fall prevention, and improved cognitive function.[36]

Clinicians should ask older adults about current levels of physical activity as part of the geriatric assessment and recommend 150 minutes of multimodal exercise. For patients with physical and medical limitations, an exercise regimen can be tailored to their needs; even smaller amounts of physical activity have been shown to have health benefits.[35]

Social assessment

The social assessment of an older adult should include information about the older adult's living situation, available support services (such as home health aides), and social network, including emergency contacts or legal power of attorney. Adequate social support is important for health because it can improve the management of chronic disease and decrease hospital utilization.[2]

As they age, approximately 90% of older adults remain in their own homes. Of those living in the community, about one-third liveS independently.[37] Thus, a comprehensive geriatric assessment should include an evaluation of the older adult's home environment and safety. If concerns are detected, home safety evaluations can be requested and performed by local home care agencies. It is also important to consider any social or financial hardships that may place patients at risk. Suspicions of abuse or neglect should be reported to the local agency on aging.

Driving

Older adults are at higher risk of automobile accidents because of a variety of conditions that are more prevalent in older age. Some states require clinicians to report to their local department of motor vehicles if there is an older adult about whom they have concerns for unsafe driving. Conditions that affect an older adult's ability to drive may include visual impairment, hearing impairment, cognitive impairment, physical disability, and medication use. Recognizing their own limitations, many older adults may independently opt to modify their driving patterns. Some may choose to only drive short distances, to avoid highways or high traffic areas, or to only drive during daylight hours.[38]

For those who continue to drive, the clinician should ask about automobile accidents and screen for conditions that may hinder an older adult's ability to drive safely. An evaluation of driving safety should begin with asking the older adult about history of automobile accidents. The clinician may wish to engage family members in this discussion. Asking a family member whether they feel comfortable riding with the older driver can often yield useful information. If concern is present, the clinician should consider any pertinent medical history and review medications in detail. Physical examination should focus on visual acuity, range of motion, and balance. Cognitive testing may identify cognitive impairment and executive dysfunction, although results have not been shown to consistently correlate with driver safety and must be interpreted in context.[39]

Because many older adults depend on driving to maintain their independence, it is important to recognize that the recommendation that a patient discontinue driving may be a difficult conversation. For older adults, relinquishing the ability to drive has been associated with a loss of independence and depression.[38] In cases whereby there is question of a driver's ability, older adults may be referred for formal driving evaluation. These assessments are conducted by trained occupational therapists, who can confirm unsafe driving habits or offer modifications to enhance driving safety.

Goals, values, and advance care planning

Understanding a patient's goals and values is a critical part of a geriatric assessment and should be used to guide further discussions about medical testing and treatment. Typically, providers consider "advance care planning" to reflect "code status" or "do-not-resuscitate" wishes, but in actuality, a broader, clearer understanding of a patient's priorities for their life and health can be vital for providers who care for them. "What brings you joy?" may be a helpful question to ask of older adults so that clinicians can begin to learn about their patients' lives and well-being outside of the medical setting.

Advance care planning involves a patient planning for future health care decisions in the event that he or she becomes incapacitated. Clinicians should aid in this process by helping patients understand their illnesses and treatment options, discussing a patient's values and goals, and eliciting treatment preferences.[40] Patients should be encouraged to include family and/or friends in these discussions and to identify a health care proxy or surrogate decision maker. Discussion of advanced directives (such as "do-not-resuscitate" status) has been shown to improve end-of-life care.

Overall, advance care planning has been associated with lower rates of in-hospital death and hospice use.[41] Prioritizing patients' values and goals, and taking into consideration their spiritual and emotional well-being, especially in the face of challenging medical decisions, can provide clarity for practitioners and ensure that patients' needs are being appropriately met.

SUMMARY

By 2030, the population older than 65 years will double to 72 million (20% of the total US population).[42] Primary care and hospital-based providers will be on the front line in the care of the growing population of older adults. A thorough review of acute and chronic medical concerns should be prioritized and considered within the context of common geriatric syndromes. A geriatric assessment evaluating cognition, function, mood, social and environmental factors, and goals of care, combined with the traditional review of systems, can help identify needs and improve the medical care and quality of life of older adults. By understanding that a comprehensive geriatric assessment can be complex and time consuming, these domains may be addressed longitudinally over a series of visits and may be enhanced by the input of interdisciplinary team members.

DISCLOSURE

The authors have nothing to disclose.

REFERENCES

1. Ellis G, Gardner M, Tsiachristas A, et al. Comprehensive geriatric assessment for older adults admitted to hospital. Cochrane Database Syst Rev 2017;2017(9). https://doi.org/10.1002/14651858.CD006211.pub3.
2. Seematter-Bagnoud L, Büla C. Brief assessments and screening for geriatric conditions in older primary care patients: a pragmatic approach. Public Health Rev 2018;39(1):8.
3. Williams TF. Comprehensive functional assessment: an overview. J Am Geriatr Soc 1983;31(11):637–41.
4. Keeler E, Guralnik JM, Tian H, et al. The impact of functional status on life expectancy in older persons. J Gerontol A Biol Sci Med Sci 2010;65A(7):727–33.
5. Elsawy B, Higgins KE. The geriatric assessment. Am Fam Physician 2011;83(1):48–56.
6. Quinn TJ, McArthur K, Ellis G, et al. Functional assessment in older people. BMJ 2011;343(aug22 1):d4681.
7. Summary of the Updated American Geriatrics Society/British Geriatrics Society Clinical Practice guideline for prevention of falls in older persons. J Am Geriatr Soc 2011;59(1):148–57.
8. Lusardi MM, Fritz S, Middleton A, et al. Determining risk of falls in community dwelling older adults: a systematic review and meta-analysis using posttest probability. J Geriatr Phys Ther 2017;40(1):1–36.
9. Studenski S, Perera S, Patel K, et al. Gait speed and survival in older adults. JAMA 2011;305(1):50–8.
10. Borson S, Scanlan JM, Chen P, et al. The Mini-Cog as a screen for dementia: validation in a population-based sample. J Am Geriatr Soc 2003;51(10):1451–4.
11. Tombaugh TN, McIntyre NJ. The mini-mental state examination: a comprehensive review. J Am Geriatr Soc 1992;40(9):922–35.

12. Nasreddine ZS, Phillips NA, Bédirian V, et al. The Montreal Cognitive Assessment, MoCA: a brief screening tool for mild cognitive impairment. J Am Geriatr Soc 2005;53(4):695–9.

13. Tariq SH, Tumosa N, Chibnall JT, et al. Comparison of the Saint Louis University mental status examination and the mini-mental state examination for detecting dementia and mild neurocognitive disorder—a pilot study. Am J Geriatr Psychiatry 2006;14(11):900–10.

14. Marcantonio ER. Delirium in hospitalized older adults. N Engl J Med 2017; 377(15):1456–66.

15. Inouye SK, van Dyck CH, Alessi CA, et al. Clarifying confusion: the confusion assessment method. A new method for detection of delirium. Ann Intern Med 1990;113(12):941–8.

16. Grover S, Kate N. Assessment scales for delirium: a review. World J Psychiatry 2012;2(4):58–70.

17. Brown EL, Raue P, Halpert KD, et al. Evidence-based guideline detection of depression in older adults with dementia. J Gerontol Nurs 2009;35(2):11–5.

18. Charney DS, Reynolds CF, Lewis L, et al. Depression and Bipolar Support Alliance consensus statement on the unmet needs in diagnosis and treatment of mood disorders in late life. Arch Gen Psychiatry 2003;60(7):664–72.

19. Siu AL, US Preventive Services Task Force (USPSTF), Bibbins-Domingo K, et al. Screening for depression in adults: US Preventive Services Task Force recommendation statement. JAMA 2016;315(4):380–7.

20. Richardson TM, He H, Podgorski C, et al. Screening for depression in aging services clients. Am J Geriatr Psychiatry 2010;18(12):1116–23.

21. Yesavage JA, Brink TL, Rose TL, et al. Development and validation of a geriatric depression screening scale: a preliminary report. J Psychiatr Res 1982;17(1): 37–49.

22. Lin FR. Hearing loss and cognition among older adults in the United States. J Gerontol A Biol Sci Med Sci 2011;66A(10):1131–6.

23. Gurgel RK, Ward PD, Schwartz S, et al. Relationship of hearing loss and dementia: a prospective, population-based study. Otol Neurotol 2014;35(5):775–81.

24. Kaiser MJ, Bauer JM, Ramsch C, et al. Validation of the Mini Nutritional Assessment short-form (MNA-SF): a practical tool for identification of nutritional status. J Nutr Health Aging 2009;13(9):782–8.

25. Kruizenga HM, Seidell JC, de Vet HCW, et al. Development and validation of a hospital screening tool for malnutrition: the short nutritional assessment questionnaire (SNAQ). Clin Nutr 2005;24(1):75–82.

26. Suskind AM, Dunn RL, Morgan DM, et al. A screening tool for clinically relevant urinary incontinence. Neurourol Urodyn 2015;34(4):332–5.

27. Maher RL, Hanlon JT, Hajjar ER. Clinical consequences of polypharmacy in elderly. Expert Opin Drug Saf 2014;13(1). https://doi.org/10.1517/14740338. 2013.827660.

28. By the 2019 American Geriatrics Society Beers Criteria® Update Expert Panel. American Geriatrics Society 2019 Updated AGS Beers Criteria® for potentially inappropriate medication use in older adults. J Am Geriatr Soc 2019;67(4): 674–94.

29. O'Mahony D, O'Sullivan D, Byrne S, et al. STOPP/START criteria for potentially inappropriate prescribing in older people: version 2. Age Ageing 2015;44(2): 213–8.

30. Anderson K, Jue SG, Madaras-Kelly KJ. Identifying patients at risk for medication mismanagement: using cognitive screens to predict a patient's accuracy in filling a pillbox. Consult Pharm 2008;23(6):459–72.

31. Society of General Internal Medicine | Choosing Wisely. Available at: https://www.choosingwisely.org/societies/society-of-general-internal-medicine/. Accessed February 13, 2020.

32. Schoenborn NL, Bowman TL, Cayea D, et al. Primary care practitioners' views on incorporating long-term prognosis in the care of older adults. JAMA Intern Med 2016;176(5):671–8.

33. Schoenborn NL, Lee K, Pollack CE, et al. Older adults' views and communication preferences about cancer screening cessation. JAMA Intern Med 2017;177(8):1121–8.

34. Kim DK, Hunter P. Advisory committee on immunization practices recommended immunization schedule for adults aged 19 years or older - United States, 2019. MMWR Morb Mortal Wkly Rep 2019;68(5):115–8.

35. Piercy KL, Troiano RP, Ballard RM, et al. The physical activity guidelines for Americans. JAMA 2018;320(19):2020–8.

36. Elsawy B, Higgins KE. Physical activity guidelines for older adults. Am Fam Physician 2010;81(1):55–9.

37. Institute on Aging | Information on Senior Citizens Living in America. Inst Aging. Available at: https://www.ioaging.org/aging-in-america. Accessed February 2, 2020.

38. Betz ME, Lowenstein SR. Driving patterns of older adults: results from the second injury control and risk survey. J Am Geriatr Soc 2010;58(10):1931–5.

39. Bennett JM, Chekaluk E, Batchelor J. Cognitive tests and determining fitness to drive in dementia: a systematic review. J Am Geriatr Soc 2016;64(9):1904–17.

40. Detering KM, Hancock AD, Reade MC, et al. The impact of advance care planning on end of life care in elderly patients: randomised controlled trial. BMJ 2010;340. https://doi.org/10.1136/bmj.c1345.

41. Bischoff KE, Sudore R, Miao Y, et al. Advance care planning and the quality of end-of-life care among older adults. J Am Geriatr Soc 2013;61(2). https://doi.org/10.1111/jgs.12105.

42. Ortman JM, Velkoff VA, Hogan H. An Aging Nation: The Older Population in the United States. Hyattsville, MD: US Census Bureau; 2014.

The Intersection of Falls and Dementia in Primary Care
Evaluation and Management Considerations

Colleen M. Casey, PhD, ANP-BC[a],*, Jamie Caulley, DPT[a],
Elizabeth A. Phelan, MD, MS[b]

KEYWORDS

- Falls • Fall prevention • Older adults • Persons with dementia
- Rehabilitation services • Risk assessment and management • Physical therapy
- Occupational therapy

KEY POINTS

- Often falls and dementia are considered to be discrete conditions. However, these conditions frequently co-occur, and one may precede the other.
- Visuospatial or gait changes may occur in older adults before obvious cognitive deficits. A fall, especially more than one or one resulting in injury, should prompt clinicians to evaluate a person's cognition.
- Strong evidence supports fall risk assessment and management for noncognitively impaired older adults. Evidence also suggests that persons with cognitive impairment can benefit from interventions to reduce fall risk.
- Older adults with cognitive impairment can benefit from additional approaches to fall risk reduction, including involving caregivers and proactively engaging with rehabilitation specialists trained in falls and cognitive impairment who can use modified training techniques.
- Recurrent falls or one or more injurious falls may represent an inflection point to shift the focus of care from reducing risk to a more palliative, supportive approach.

INTRODUCTION

Although a substantial body of research has characterized the burden of falls among older adults, most discussions of fall risk and interventions do not explore the trajectory of falls among populations particularly at risk, such as persons with dementia.

[a] Senior Health Program, Providence Health & Services, 4400 NE Halsey, Fifth Floor, Portland, OR 97213, USA; [b] Department of Medicine, Division of Gerontology and Geriatric Medicine, University of Washington, Harborview Medical Center, 325 9th Avenue, Box 359755, Seattle, WA 98104-2499, USA
* Corresponding author.
E-mail address: Colleen.Casey@providence.org

Med Clin N Am 104 (2020) 791–806
https://doi.org/10.1016/j.mcna.2020.06.003
0025-7125/20/© 2020 Elsevier Inc. All rights reserved.

Often falls and dementia are considered to be discrete conditions, with their evaluation and management considered separately. However, these conditions frequently co-occur, and one may precede the other. This article summarizes what is known about the relationship between falls and dementia in community-dwelling older adults. The term "cognitive impairment" refers to persons with both mild cognitive impairment (MCI) as well as dementia unless MCI or the type of dementia is specifically stated.

BACKGROUND

The burden of falls has reached epidemic proportions. Each day, 74 people aged 65 years and older die from a fall—one person every 20 minutes.[1] Approximately 30% to 40% of community-dwelling older adults fall annually, with those who are older, sicker, and more dependent falling more frequently and having a heightened mortality risk.[2] Medical care for falls costs approximately $50.0 billion annually in the United States.[3] Perhaps just as alarming is the personal cost of falling, with older adults who have fallen experiencing heightened anxiety about falling, physical deconditioning and immobility, loss of independence, and the need for a higher level of care.[4] Many older adults consider this loss of independence and psychological toll to be worse than death.

Despite there being good evidence of the effectiveness of fall risk reduction strategies to decrease fall risk by as much as 25% to 30%,[5,6] many older adults forget about a fall or diminish its significance and do not discuss their fall with their primary care provider (PCP).[7] Most PCPs report not knowing how to conduct a fall risk assessment nor how to systematically address risk once it is identified.[8]

Fortunately, the Centers for Disease Control and Prevention (CDC) have prioritized fall risk screening and management to help medical providers, their teams, and health care systems assess and manage fall risk. Based on clinical practice guidelines from the American and British Geriatrics Societies (AGS/BGS), the CDC developed the Stopping Elderly Accidents, Deaths, and Injuries (STEADI) toolkit.[8] A cornerstone of STEADI is the validated 12-item "Stay Independent" falls screening instrument (STEADI questionnaire).[9] This questionnaire identifies patients at fall risk: a score greater than or equal to 4 indicates increased risk of falling. Beyond the risk score, the STEADI questionnaire has clinical utility in that individual questions highlight certain actionable fall risk factors (eg, impaired balance). STEADI application has thus far focused on the general, community-dwelling older adult population, either explicitly excluding patients with dementia or without special regard for dementia diagnoses.[10,11]

THE BURDEN OF FALLS IN PERSONS WITH DEMENTIA

Epidemiologic research on falls among persons with dementia has found that cognitively impaired individuals have 8 to 10 times more incident falls than persons without dementia,[12] with falls being the second leading cause of hospital readmission for those with cognitive impairment.[13] Those who have dementia with prominent motor features, such as dementia with lewy bodies (DLB) and Parkinson disease dementia (PDD) are at the highest risk.[12] People with dementia are also more likely to injure[14] and less likely to recover from a fall. For example, Alzheimer type dementia (AD) confers a 3-fold increase in risk of hip fracture as well as an increased mortality rate subsequent to hip fracture.[15]

FALL RISK FACTORS IN THE GENERAL OLDER ADULT POPULATION

Multiple factors influence an older adult's fall risk, and risk increases linearly with the number of risk factors present.[2] Risk factors include, but are not limited to, history of prior falls[16,17]; age and age-related changes; female sex; autonomic dysfunction/orthostatic changes; chronic illnesses (eg, diabetes, depression); gait, strength, and balance deficits, including impaired static standing balance[18]; sensory deficits; central nervous system (CNS)-active medications; unsupportive footwear; improper assistive devices and home/environmental safety issues; behaviors/choices, such as alcohol consumption[19]; fear of falling[20]; and frailty.[21] Fall risk factors are broadly categorized as extrinsic (external to the individual) or intrinsic (within the individual) and also as modifiable or nonmodifiable,[22] with some risk factors more pronounced or unique in persons with dementia (**Fig. 1**).

FALL RISK FACTORS IN PERSONS WITH DEMENTIA
Demographic Factors

Similar to the general population, the risk of falls and injurious falls increases with age for those with dementia.[23] Women are at greater risk for falls,[24] injuries,[25] and fall-related hospitalizations[25] than men, and among persons with dementia, women are at greater risk for recurrent injurious falls resulting in hospitalization.[23]

Gait and Balance Impairments

Gait and balance impairments are common, and often more severe, in persons with dementia. Evidence suggests that changes in gait may occur very early in the disease process and may precede any detectable cognitive deficits. For example, gait variability, or fluctuations in gait characteristics (stride length, speed) from one stride to the next, is associated with a 12-fold increased risk of cognitive decline over a 4-year period among adults with previously normal cognitive testing.[26] Other studies

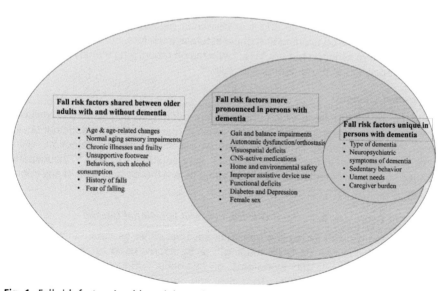

Fig. 1. Fall risk factors in older adults with and without dementia.

have also found significant associations between gait speed and cognitive changes preceding any formal diagnosis of cognitive dysfunction.[27]

Sedentary Behavior

Community-dwelling persons with dementia spend most of the time in sedentary behavior and have low levels of physical activity.[28] Compared with those who are cognitively intact, persons with dementia spend significantly more of their waking hours in a sedentary state and significantly less time in light-to-moderate and moderate-to-vigorous intensity activities.[29] A decline in executive functioning, which is necessary for goal-directed behavior, may explain the higher level of sedentary time. Inactivity leads to muscle weakness, thereby contributing to fall risk.

Autonomic Dysfunction and Orthostatic Hypotension

Autonomic dysfunction can occur as part of normal aging and result in orthostatic hypotension and syncopal episodes, affecting nearly 30% of community-dwelling older adults.[30] Persons with dementia are more likely to have orthostatic hypotension and autonomic neuropathy, with DLB and PDD having the highest prevalence.[12] An orthostatic syncopal mechanism underlies nearly half of initially unexplained falls among persons with dementia.[31] Medications that contribute to orthostatic hypotension-induced syncope among persons with dementia include nitrates, alpha-blockers, and combinations of ace-inhibitors and diuretics and ace-inhibitors and nitrates.[32]

Central Nervous System-Active Medications

For both the general older population and persons with dementia, CNS-active medications (eg, benzodiazepines, antidepressants, antipsychotics) contribute to fall risk and are widely used, including by persons with dementia.[33] Evidence suggests that older adults with dementia may be more sensitive to the effects of CNS-active medications.[34] Current use of centrally acting agents increases the risk of fall-related injuries among persons with dementia, even with use of low dosages.[35] Anticholinergic drugs increase both falls and fall-related injuries among persons with dementia, with even low-potency agents increasing fall risk when more than one is taken.[36,37] Data on the effect of dementia medications on falls are mixed, with a meta-analysis concluding that cholinesterase inhibitors, such as donepezil, increase the risk of syncope but not falls,[38] whereas a recent single study found a significant association of these agents with falls.[39]

Visuospatial Changes

In addition to aging-related vision changes (eg, decreased acuity, color sensitivity, depth perception), persons with cognitive deficits may experience additional oculovisual changes including diminished contrast sensitivity, motion detection, visual fields, and visuospatial function, all of which may contribute to falls.[40] Visuospatial changes have been detected as early as 3 years before the identification of any cognitive changes.[41]

Severity of Dementia, Behavioral Disturbance, and Functional Decline

Fall risk increases with increasing dementia severity, either as determined by white matter cortical changes on CNS imaging[18] or by scores used to characterize the severity of neuropsychiatric symptoms of dementia.[42] Behavioral disturbances, including wandering,[43] verbally disruptive and attention-seeking behaviors, and impulsivity contribute to fall risk in those with dementia.[18] There is also evidence that wandering may stem, in part, from unmet needs, which are highly prevalent among persons with dementia.[44]

As dementia progresses, function typically declines. Greater dependence in basic activities of daily living (ADL) has been identified as an independent risk factor for falling among persons with and without dementia.[14,16,17]

Reduced Safety Awareness and Fear of Falling

As part of the dementia disease process, cognitive processing slows; attention and executive function decline; ability to multi-task declines; judgment worsens; and deficits in motor planning prevent a person from adapting their gait appropriately to changes in the environment. These changes lead to reduced safety awareness, with declines in cognitive flexibility diminishing a person's ability to quickly respond to changes in the external environment, such as adjustments for an oncoming car, a slippery walkway, new or unexpected curb cuts, or construction.[45]

Fear of falling is a known risk factor in the general older adult population. Older adults with mild cognitive impairment more often reported a fear of falling and scored higher in their concern for falling than their counterparts with AD, likely reflecting a gradual loss of insight and judgment following dementia onset.[46]

Comorbidities

Certain comorbidities have been found to increase the risk of falls for those with and without cognitive impairment, which include diabetes and depression. Persons with dementia who have comorbid diabetes may be more susceptible to hypoglycemia and subsequent adverse events such as falls and fractures.[17,47] Several studies have found depression to be an independent risk factor for falls in persons with mild-to-moderate dementia,[12,16,18,48] even after adjustment for antidepressant use.[48]

Home Safety Risks

Persons with dementia who live at home have been found to have significantly more home safety hazards than their counterparts who live in an institutional setting.[49] Home hazards for community dwellers with dementia include low chairs, lack of grab bars around the toilet, toilets that are too low, loose rugs, lack of night lights, and missing railings on stairs.[49]

Caregiver Burden

Caregiver burden has been identified as a fall risk factor for community-dwelling persons with dementia.[18] Higher caregiver burden scores are associated with falls and fracture, suggesting that caregiver distress may contribute to fall risk.[50,51] Caregiver anxiety was the measure most closely tied to patient fracture risk and represents a potentially modifiable fall risk factor.[51]

FALL RISK ASSESSMENT IN THE GENERAL OLDER ADULT POPULATION

The basics of a comprehensive fall risk assessment are well documented and include taking a thorough falls history; conducting a medication review to identify CNS-active medications; performing a falls-focused physical examination; and discussing functional and environment risk factors.[22,52] Using a standardized screening tool, such as the STEADI Stay Independent questionnaire (available at https://www.cdc.gov/steadi/pdf/STEADI-Brochure-StayIndependent-508.pdf), helps to identify particular risk factors and direct interventions.[9] Key components of the physical examination include orthostatic vital signs to screen for postural hypotension; visual acuity and peripheral vision; a cardiac examination; evaluation of gait and balance; functional lower extremity strength and sensation; and a foot examination.

Cognitive screening is also an important part of a fall-related evaluation, particularly after someone has fallen.[22] Among almost 350 community-dwelling adults, aged 75 years and older, receiving care through a large health care system, cognitive screening done as part of routine care after a single fall-related emergency room visit identified cognitive impairment in nearly half (48%) of the sample.[53] This, combined with the understanding that changes in gait often precede onset of MCI and dementia, supports completion of a brief cognitive screen, such as the Mini-Cog,[54] as part of the falls-focused examination.

FALL RISK ASSESSMENT UNIQUE TO PERSONS WITH DEMENTIA

The standard approach for fall risk assessment serves as the foundation for any fall risk assessment in older adults with dementia. To the authors' knowledge, there is no validated fall risk screening tool specifically tailored for persons with dementia living in the community. Because three-quarters of persons with dementia live with someone in their home,[55] the authors recommend enlisting the primary caregiver of the person with dementia or someone who knows the person well to help complete the STEADI Stay Independent questionnaire. The caregiver can also provide a history of the person's exercise habits and daily routines as well as their functional status.

The falls-focused physical examination remains an important assessment, especially for persons with dementia. Particular attention should be given to the cardiac evaluation and assessment for orthostasis, given the increased risk of autonomic dysfunction and syncope in persons with dementia.[31] A thorough review of medications, including over-the-counter medications, identifying those that are CNS-active and/or might contribute to orthostatic hypotension is also critical. Updating the eye examination to ensure that preventable causes of vision loss (eg, cataract, glaucoma) are identified and managed is important, because a person with dementia may not spontaneously report vision changes.

The assessment of gait, strength, and balance using standardized tests with individuals with cognitive limitations may be challenging. However, gait speed holds promise for fall risk screening in people with dementia and requires little instruction.[56] Simple tests of strength and balance that are part of the STEADI approach (ie, chair stand and 4-stage balance test, at https://www.cdc.gov/steadi/materials.html) are still feasible to assess, even with persons with advanced dementia, by demonstrating each test first and asking the patient to mimic the demonstration. A foot examination not only provides meaningful information about structural deformities and neuropathy that may adversely affect balance but can also help with assessing self-care (ADL) ability by observing whether a person is able to don and doff their shoes independently.

REDUCING FALL RISK THROUGH INTERVENTIONS IN THE GENERAL OLDER ADULT POPULATION

Evidence has consistently supported exercise and the targeted use of multifactorial interventions to reduce fall risk in cognitively intact older adults.[5,57] A recent network meta-analysis[6] found exercise alone, and exercise combined with other interventions such as vision, with or without environmental modification, to be effective in preventing injurious falls.

A systematic review of the effect of exercise on fall risk found that high-dosage exercise ($\geq$50 hours accumulated over a minimum of 25 weeks), with a focus on balance training, and no walking program, reduced fall risk by an average of 17%.[58] These findings are consistent with those of a randomized trial showing that walking alone, absent any balance or strengthening program, was not effective in reducing falls.[59] Tai Chi participation has been shown to decrease falls by as much as 50% when practiced twice weekly for 24 weeks.[60]

Data on vitamin D supplementation have been more mixed, with some studies suggesting a high dose being associated with more fall-related outcomes.[61] The United States Preventive Services Task Force recently adopted formal recommendations, based on a separate review, supporting exercise but not vitamin D supplementation to prevent falls in at-risk community-dwelling adults aged 65 years or older.[62] However, these recommendations do not apply to those with osteoporosis, at increased risk of falls, or vitamin D deficiency. Given that many community-dwelling older adults have or are at risk for osteoporosis, vitamin D3 intake of at least 4000 IU daily across all sources is still appropriate for many older adults on this basis, without the need for first checking vitamin D levels.[63]

Other modifiable risk factors that can be prioritized with community-dwelling older adults at fall risk include dose reduction and/or elimination of CNS-active medications (also see STEADI-Rx at https://www.cdc.gov/steadi/steadi-rx.html),[64] single lens glasses for distance wear with those who routinely exercise outdoors,[65] addressing home safety hazards through home modification,[66] and podiatric interventions for those with foot pain.[67]

THE ROLE OF REHABILITATION IN PREVENTION OF FALLS
Older Adults with Normal Cognition

For older adults at increased risk of falling who have gait, strength, and balance impairments, rehabilitation services (physical therapy and/or occupational therapy) are recommended to help address modifiable fall risk factors and improve physical performance to enable successful participation in home- or community-based exercise on a long-term basis.[68] Physical therapists (PTs) can focus therapy on balance retraining; evaluating and managing dizziness; assessing appropriateness of an assistive device; and designing an individualized progressive and sustainable long-term exercise regimen that includes balance and strength exercises. Occupational therapists (OTs) can attend to functional deficits affecting mobility, ADL modification to reduce fall risk–taking behaviors, home safety modifications, and adaptive device provision and training.[69] Home safety assessments with follow-up modifications have been demonstrated to decrease fall risk from 19% to 34%[5,66] and are particularly effective for those at high risk of falls.[5] Whether through regular multimodal exercise, such as Tai Chi, or from exercises prescribed by rehabilitation specialists, it is important to remember that the benefits of these activities persist only as long as the person continues with the program.

Despite a clear role for PTs and OTs in fall prevention, rehabilitation specific to falls and fall-related injuries may be underutilized. Only 50% of patients identified at high risk of falls receive fall-related rehabilitation services.[68] Even for at-risk patients seen by PTs or OTs, only a minority had falls explicitly addressed during rehabilitation.[68]

Because gait impairments can precede cognitive deficits and any diagnosis of MCI or dementia, PTs and OTs can play an important role in alerting the health care team of any concerning changes in gait. In fact, an estimated 11% to 18% of patients in rehabilitation services with moderate-to-high fall risk were determined to have possible or probable dementia, suggesting that therapists are already seeing these patients in their practices.[68]

Older Adults with Cognitive Impairment

Systematic reviews have also confirmed the benefit of exercise for fall risk reduction among community-dwelling persons with mild-to-moderate dementia.[37,70–72] Exercise programs are generally multimodal (strength, balance, and aerobic components), designed or supervised by a PT, and performed at least 2 to 3 times per week for a minimum of at least 25 weeks.[70] Many involve the caregiver of the person living with dementia.[70,71] Exercise interventions have been found to slow the rate of functional loss in the early stages of cognitive decline, with a protective effect against falls in advanced stages.[72] Importantly, home-based physical activity programs may also reduce caregiver burden, a risk factor for falls in this population.[73]

A limited number of studies of Tai Chi are underway with persons with dementia.[74–76] Results from these studies are not yet available; early results suggest that Tai Chi is feasible, especially when a caregiver is involved.[74,76] Caregivers can play a key role in helping an older adult with dementia structure their day to include physical activity.

COGNITIVE TRAINING

Cognitive training, using specific exercises to increase neural plasticity, can target specific cognitive domains associated with fall risk, such as executive function, working memory, and alternating attention. Computerized training of executive function tasks has been found to limit decline in timed up-and-go performance among cognitively intact older adults.[77] Studies in cognitively impaired older adults combining cognitive and physical interventions have also shown positive effects on balance, gait speed, and function as compared with controls but have not consistently demonstrated decreased fall rates, a finding thought to be related to heterogeneous study design.[78]

FUNCTIONAL TRAINING

Less well studied has been the role of OTs or PTs in assisting persons with dementia to increase their independence with ADLs as a means to reduce fall risk.[14,16] OT-driven interventions increase function and independence, but fall risk reduction has not been specifically measured.[79] A complete functional history of past activities and hobbies of persons with dementia may guide therapists in tailoring strategies that call on procedural memory, which is preserved even as dementia progresses.[80] Examples of preserved procedural memory in relation to ADL function include standing up from a seated position, climbing stairs, tying a shoe, and brushing one's teeth.

ERRORLESS LEARNING

Persons with cognitive deficits may benefit from alternative training approaches. Errorless learning can be used by therapists and other clinicians when a person with cognitive impairment demonstrates an inability to learn using the traditional trial and error approach, a common learning strategy among cognitively intact individuals.[80] Errorless learning, a teaching style used across therapeutic disciplines, has been shown to be effective in teaching skills to adults with cognitive impairment to increase independence, function, and safety.[81] In errorless learning, the therapist sets up a task in order to reduce the opportunity for errors and guessing. The task (eg, standing up safely from a chair) is practiced with the same consistent structure each time until the learner excels at the task, at which point structured cues are gradually removed. Errorless learning has been used in ADL training, mobility training, and in communication skills training.[81]

PRESCRIPTION AND SAFE USE OF MOBILITY AIDS

PTs and OTs are trained to assess suitability of assistive devices for persons with and without cognitive impairment. The use of a walker, cane, or other mobility device can support trunk or lower limb weakness, unload painful joints, or offer a wider base of support, but the person must be able to operate the device safely. As executive function and attentional control decline with the progression of dementia, a person's energy "cost" to use these devices increases. In the case of new device users, a slower and more challenging gait may result.[82] In some cases, an inappropriate device can actually increase a person's risk of falling.[83]

It is clear that persons with dementia require different approaches in their exercise and rehabilitation, suggesting that identifying rehabilitation professionals experienced in working with these individuals will maximize the likelihood of reducing fall risk. Clinicians should be versed in the various types and stages of dementia, trained to apply alternative learning techniques, and experienced and willing to involve a caregiver in the rehabilitation process.

REDUCING FALL RISK THROUGH OTHER INTERVENTIONS IN PERSONS WITH DEMENTIA

Given the heightened risk of falling of persons with dementia, it is imperative that PCPs proactively assess and tailor fall risk interventions for known modifiable risk factors for their patients with cognitive impairment. In addition to the focus on strength, balance, and rehabilitation activities described earlier, management of orthostatic hypotension, early intervention for first cataract,[40] tapering or eliminating use of CNS-active medications when safe and appropriate, preventing hypoglycemia, and treating comorbid depression are reasonable targets for intervention.[12,47,84] Although there is a dearth of trial evidence for interventions targeting fall risk factors specific to person with dementia (eg, behavioral disturbances; unmet needs such as thirst, hunger, pain), addressing these risk factors through evidence-based interventions[85] may also help reduce falls and injuries (**Fig. 2**).

WHEN RESTORATIVE REHABILITATION IS NO LONGER THE GOAL

Rehabilitation therapists can help recognize when it might be appropriate to shift the focus from progressive improvement-based rehabilitation to a more palliative approach that focuses on preserving or improving functional capacity with an emphasis on quality of life. Along the spectrum of older adults with dementia who fall are those who have recurrent falls, fall-related hospitalizations, one or more injurious falls, or become increasingly frail. Once a person with dementia has progressed to a point of significantly diminished functional capacity and compromised quality of life, such as in stage 7 of the Functional Assessment Staging of Alzheimer's Disease scale,[86] it is reasonable to frame management of fall risk in a different light.[86] At this point, falls can represent an inflection point, an opportunity to evaluate falls in the context of the person's overall health, functional status, and disease process, with less focus on reversing fall risk factors.[87] To date, this area is understudied. Based on their clinical experiences, for this stage of care, the authors recommend educating caregivers that falls are intrinsic to dementia's progression, as well as addressing functional needs, caregiving support, and de-escalating medical management for chronic conditions.[43]

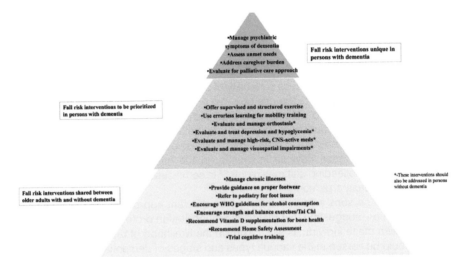

Fig. 2. Fall risk interventions in older adults with and without dementia. CNS, central nervous system; WHO, World Health Organization.[a] These interventions should also be addressed in persons without dementia.

SUMMARY

The assessment and management of fall risk is a critical focus for preventive care in the primary care setting with all older adults, both those with and without cognitive impairment. The idea that falls and fall risk be regarded as a chronic condition that deserves longitudinal attention by PCPs and their care teams[22] is particularly relevant for those with progressive neurodegenerative disorders. Although validated tools to assess fall risk in persons with cognitive impairment are currently lacking, the STEADI Stay Independent questionnaire is a presently available option and can be completed by caregivers of persons with dementia.

The evidence presented herein justifies PCPs in recommending exercise, with strength and balance components, for all their older adult patients, including those with cognitive deficits. Exercise seems to be an effective approach to fall prevention in those with dementia, even across the spectrum of disease severity. Balance and strength exercises, practiced with the support of a caregiver for a minimum of at least 25 weeks,[74,76] can reduce falls[70,72] and also improve overall functional status.[72] For patients who need more targeted help, PCPs can recommend and refer their patients to PTs and OTs for rehabilitation and recommend optimizing the safety of the home environment. Early referral to rehabilitation, when a person is less cognitively impaired and at a lower fall risk, allows the individual to gain the most from rehabilitation services.

More limited evidence exists for addressing other fall risk factors in persons with cognitive impairment. Even so, it is imperative to avoid therapeutic nihilism by promulgating the idea that falls are universally part of "normal" aging, regardless of cognitive status. This view leads to the undertreatment of falls, just as it does the undertreatment of other diseases disproportionately experienced by older adults, such as cancer.[88]

With the awareness that gait and visuospatial changes can precede any obvious signs of cognitive impairment, PCPs should remain alert when a patient has gait or vision changes, especially when accompanied by a fall.[89] A fall event can serve as an opportunity to assess for cognitive impairment. Using a fall-related diagnostic code (eg, history of fall), along with a code to indicate the presence of cognitive impairment, can alert rehabilitation colleagues to focus on fall risk while taking into consideration a person's underlying cognitive deficits.

The authors suggest shifting to a more palliative approach to falls when patients reach the more advanced stages of dementia and are unable to participate in exercise and/or no longer seem to be deriving any benefit from fall risk reduction efforts. At this point, the PCP and team can work with the patient, family, and caregivers to reframe the conversation about falls to facilitate care that optimizes the safety, comfort, and well-being of the person with dementia.

CLINICS CARE POINTS

- There is strong evidence supporting assessment and management of modifiable fall risk factors for noncognitively impaired older adults who screen positive for fall risk based on validated screening tools.
- Evidence also suggests that patients with cognitive impairment may benefit from fall risk reduction interventions, in particular exercise aimed at optimizing strength and balance.
- Therapeutic nihilism should be avoided with all older adults, including those with cognitive impairment, who are very old, and those with prior falls, as they can still benefit from fall prevention exercise programs.
- Particular considerations in managing fall risk with older adults who have cognitive impairment include involvement of a caregiver and rehabilitation specialists who can use modified training techniques.
- A fall, changes in gait, and/or changes in visual function may be harbingers of cognitive decline and present an opportunity for early attention and intervention to target fall risk factors.
- In patients with advanced dementia who are unable to engage in fall risk reduction (eg, exercise), a shift in focus from risk factor reduction to a more palliative, supportive approach may be appropriate.

DISCLOSURE

This work was not directly funded by any grant. However, it was indirectly funded through other work by the Institute for Healthcare Improvement and the John A. Hartford Foundation, which funded our organization's Age Friendly Health System work. For the JAHF, they funded both an Age-Friendly Health System grant (Casey/Caulley) as well as through a Practice Change Leader's grant (Casey). The Practice Change Leader grant was also funded through Atlantic Philanthropies.

REFERENCES

1. Centers for Disease Control and Prevention. Older adult falls: a growing danger. 2020. Available at: https://www.cdc.gov/steadi/pdf/STEADI_MediaFactSheet-a. pdf. Accessed January 29, 2020.

2. Tinetti ME, Speechley M, Ginter SF. Risk factors for falls among elderly persons living in the community. N Engl J Med 1988;319(26):1701–7.

3. Florence CS, Bergen G, Atherly A, et al. Medical costs of fatal and nonfatal falls in older adults. J Am Geriatr Soc 2018;66(4):693–8.

4. Hadjistavropoulos T, Martin RR, Sharpe D, et al. A longitudinal investigation of fear of falling, fear of pain, and activity avoidance in community-dwelling older adults. J Aging Health 2007;19(6):965–84.

5. Gillespie LD, Robertson MC, Gillespie WJ, et al. Interventions for preventing falls in older people living in the community. Cochrane Database Syst Rev 2012;(9):CD007146.

6. Tricco AC, Thomas SM, Veroniki AA, et al. Comparisons of interventions for preventing falls in older adults: a systematic review and meta-analysis. JAMA 2017; 318(17):1687–99.

7. Stevens JA, Ballesteros MF, Mack KA, et al. Gender differences in seeking care for falls in the aged Medicare population. Am J Prev Med 2012;43(1):59–62.

8. Stevens JA, Phelan EA. Development of STEADI: a fall prevention resource for health care providers. Health Promot Pract 2013;14(5):706–14.

9. Rubenstein LZ, Vivrette R, Harker JO, et al. Validating an evidence-based, self-rated fall risk questionnaire (FRQ) for older adults. J Safety Res 2011;42(6): 493–9.

10. Eckstrom E, Parker EM, Lambert GH, et al. Implementing STEADI in academic primary care to address older adult fall risk. Innov Aging 2017;1(2):igx028.

11. Johnston YA, Bergen G, Bauer M, et al. Implementation of the stopping elderly accidents, deaths, and injuries initiative in primary care: an outcome evaluation. Gerontologist 2019;59(6):1182–91.

12. Allan LM, Ballard CG, Rowan EN, et al. Incidence and prediction of falls in dementia: a prospective study in older people. PLoS One 2009;4(5):e5521.

13. Hoffman GJ, Liu H, Alexander NB, et al. Posthospital fall injuries and 30-day readmissions in adults 65 years and older. JAMA Netw Open 2019;2(5):e194276.

14. Ek S, Rizzuto D, Fratiglioni L, et al. Risk profiles for injurious falls in people over 60: a population-based cohort study. J Gerontol A Biol Sci Med Sci 2018;73(2): 233–9.

15. Baker NL, Cook MN, Arrighi HM, et al. Hip fracture risk and subsequent mortality among Alzheimer's disease patients in the United Kingdom, 1988-2007. Age Ageing 2011;40(1):49–54.

16. Salva A, Roque M, Rojano X, et al. Falls and risk factors for falls in community-dwelling adults with dementia (NutriAlz trial). Alzheimer Dis Assoc Disord 2012; 26(1):74–80.

17. Perttila NM, Ohman H, Strandberg TE, et al. How do community-dwelling persons with Alzheimer Disease fall? Falls in the FINALEX study. Dement Geriatr Cogn Dis Extra 2017;7(2):195–203.

18. Fernando E, Fraser M, Hendriksen J, et al. Risk factors associated with falls in older adults with dementia: a systematic review. Physiother Can 2017;69(2): 161–70.

19. Panel on Prevention of Falls in Older Persons. Summary of the Updated American Geriatrics Society/British Geriatrics Society clinical practice guideline for prevention of falls in older persons. J Am Geriatr Soc 2011;59(1):148–57.

20. Friedman SM, Munoz B, West SK, et al. Falls and fear of falling: which comes first? A longitudinal prediction model suggests strategies for primary and secondary prevention. J Am Geriatr Soc 2002;50(8):1329–35.

21. Cheng MH, Chang SF. Frailty as a risk factor for falls among community dwelling people: evidence from a meta-analysis. J Nurs Scholarsh 2017;49(5):529–36.

22. Phelan EA, Mahoney JE, Voit JC, et al. Assessment and management of fall risk in primary care settings. Med Clin North Am 2015;99(2):281–93.

23. Meuleners LB, Fraser ML, Bulsara MK, et al. Risk factors for recurrent injurious falls that require hospitalization for older adults with dementia: a population based study. BMC Neurol 2016;16(1):188.
24. Deandrea S, Lucenteforte E, Bravi F, et al. Risk factors for falls in community-dwelling older people: a systematic review and meta-analysis. Epidemiology 2010;21(5):658–68.
25. Stevens JA, Sogolow ED. Gender differences for non-fatal unintentional fall related injuries among older adults. Inj Prev 2005;11(2):115–9.
26. Byun S, Han JW, Kim TH, et al. Gait variability can predict the risk of cognitive decline in cognitively normal older people. Dement Geriatr Cogn Disord 2018; 45(5–6):251–61.
27. Grande G, Triolo F, Nuara A, et al. Measuring gait speed to better identify prodromal dementia. Exp Gerontol 2019;124:110625.
28. van Alphen HJ, Volkers KM, Blankevoort CG, et al. Older adults with dementia are sedentary for most of the day. PLoS One 2016;11(3):e0152457.
29. Hartman YAW, Karssemeijer EGA, van Diepen LAM, et al. Dementia patients are more sedentary and less physically active than age- and sex-matched cognitively healthy older adults. Dement Geriatr Cogn Disord 2018;46(1–2):81–9.
30. Kamaruzzaman S, Watt H, Carson C, et al. The association between orthostatic hypotension and medication use in the British Women's Heart and Health Study. Age Ageing 2010;39(1):51–6.
31. Ungar A, Mussi C, Ceccofiglio A, et al. Etiology of syncope and unexplained falls in elderly adults with dementia: Syncope and Dementia (SYD) Study. J Am Geriatr Soc 2016;64(8):1567–73.
32. Testa G, Ceccofiglio A, Mussi C, et al. Hypotensive drugs and syncope due to orthostatic hypotension in older adults with dementia (Syncope and Dementia Study). J Am Geriatr Soc 2018;66(8):1532–7.
33. Tolppanen AM, Taipale H, Tanskanen A, et al. Comparison of predictors of hip fracture and mortality after hip fracture in community-dwellers with and without Alzheimer's disease - exposure-matched cohort study. BMC Geriatr 2016; 16(1):204.
34. Sunderland T, Tariot PN, Cohen RM, et al. Anticholinergic sensitivity in patients with dementia of the Alzheimer type and age-matched controls. A dose-response study. Arch Gen Psychiatry 1987;44(5):418–26.
35. Hart LA, Marcum ZA, Gray SL, et al. The association between central nervous system-active medication use and fall-related injury in community-dwelling older adults with dementia. Pharmacotherapy 2019;39(5):530–43.
36. Green AR, Reifler LM, Bayliss EA, et al. Drugs contributing to anticholinergic burden and risk of fall or fall-related injury among older adults with mild cognitive impairment, dementia and multiple chronic conditions: a retrospective cohort study. Drugs Aging 2019;36(3):289–97.
37. Perttila NM, Ohman H, Strandberg TE, et al. Effect of exercise on drug-related falls among persons with Alzheimer's Disease: a secondary analysis of the FI-NALEX study. Drugs Aging 2018;35(11):1017–23.
38. Kim DH, Brown RT, Ding EL, et al. Dementia medications and risk of falls, syncope, and related adverse events: meta-analysis of randomized controlled trials. J Am Geriatr Soc 2011;59(6):1019–31.
39. Epstein NU, Guo R, Farlow MR, et al. Medication for Alzheimer's disease and associated fall hazard: a retrospective cohort study from the Alzheimer's Disease Neuroimaging Initiative. Drugs Aging 2014;31(2):125–9.

40. Armstrong R, Kergoat H. Oculo-visual changes and clinical considerations affecting older patients with dementia. Ophthalmic Physiol Opt 2015;35(4): 352–76.
41. Johnson DK, Storandt M, Morris JC, et al. Longitudinal study of the transition from healthy aging to Alzheimer disease. Arch Neurol 2009;66(10):1254–9.
42. Roitto HM, Kautiainen H, Ohman H, et al. Relationship of neuropsychiatric symptoms with falls in Alzheimer's Disease - Does exercise modify the risk? J Am Geriatr Soc 2018;66(12):2377–81.
43. Buchner DM, Larson EB. Falls and fractures in patients with Alzheimer-type dementia. JAMA 1987;257(11):1492–5.
44. Black BS, Johnston D, Rabins PV, et al. Unmet needs of community-residing persons with dementia and their informal caregivers: findings from the maximizing independence at home study. J Am Geriatr Soc 2013;61(12):2087–95.
45. Zhang W, Low LF, Schwenk M, et al. Review of gait, cognition, and fall risks with implications for fall prevention in older adults with dementia. Dement Geriatr Cogn Disord 2019;48(1–2):17–29.
46. Borges Sde M, Radanovic M, Forlenza OV. Fear of falling and falls in older adults with mild cognitive impairment and Alzheimer's disease. Neuropsychol Dev Cogn B Aging Neuropsychol Cogn 2015;22(3):312–21.
47. Mattishent K, Richardson K, Dhatariya K, et al. The effects of hypoglycaemia and dementia on cardiovascular events, falls and fractures and all-cause mortality in older individuals: a retrospective cohort study. Diabetes Obes Metab 2019;21(9): 2076–85.
48. Taylor ME, Delbaere K, Lord SR, et al. Neuropsychological, physical, and functional mobility measures associated with falls in cognitively impaired older adults. J Gerontol A Biol Sci Med Sci 2014;69(8):987–95.
49. Lowery K, Buri H, Ballard C. What is the prevalence of environmental hazards in the homes of dementia sufferers and are they associated with falls. Int J Geriatr Psychiatry 2000;15(10):883–6.
50. Kuzuya M, Masuda Y, Hirakawa Y, et al. Falls of the elderly are associated with burden of caregivers in the community. Int J Geriatr Psychiatry 2006;21(8):740–5.
51. Maggio D, Ercolani S, Andreani S, et al. Emotional and psychological distress of persons involved in the care of patients with Alzheimer disease predicts falls and fractures in their care recipients. Dement Geriatr Cogn Disord 2010;30(1):33–8.
52. Tinetti ME, Williams TF, Mayewski R. Fall risk index for elderly patients based on number of chronic disabilities. Am J Med 1986;80(3):429–34.
53. Casey CM, Kuebrich MB, Engstrom K, et al. Seniors at risk for falling after emergency room visit (SAFER): when are falls a proxy for unmet needs and frailty. Sunriver (OR): Oregon Geriatrics Society Meeting; 2019.
54. Borson S, Scanlan J, Brush M, et al. The mini-cog: a cognitive 'vital signs' measure for dementia screening in multi-lingual elderly. Int J Geriatr Psychiatry 2000; 15(11):1021–7.
55. Association As. 2019 Alzheimer's disease facts and figures. 2019. Available at: https://www.alz.org/media/documents/alzheimers-facts-and-figures-2019-r.pdf. Accessed January 29, 2020.
56. Allali G, Launay CP, Blumen HM, et al. Falls, cognitive impairment, and gait performance: results from the GOOD initiative. J Am Med Dir Assoc 2017;18(4): 335–40.
57. Moyer VA. Prevention of falls in community-dwelling older adults: U.S. Preventive Services Task Force recommendation statement. Ann Intern Med 2012;157(3): 197–204.

58. Sherrington C, Whitney JC, Lord SR, et al. Effective exercise for the prevention of falls: a systematic review and meta-analysis. J Am Geriatr Soc 2008;56(12): 2234–43.

59. Voukelatos A, Merom D, Sherrington C, et al. The impact of a home-based walking programme on falls in older people: the Easy Steps randomised controlled trial. Age Ageing 2015;44(3):377–83.

60. Li F, Harmer P, Fitzgerald K, et al. Effectiveness of a therapeutic Tai Ji Quan intervention vs a multimodal exercise intervention to prevent falls among older adults at high risk of falling: a randomized clinical trial. JAMA Intern Med 2018;178(10): 1301–10.

61. Sanders KM, Stuart AL, Williamson EJ, et al. Annual high-dose oral vitamin D and falls and fractures in older women: a randomized controlled trial. JAMA 2010; 303(18):1815–22.

62. Guirguis-Blake JM, Michael YL, Perdue LA, et al. Interventions to prevent falls in older adults: updated evidence report and systematic review for the US Preventive Services Task Force. JAMA 2018;319(16):1705–16.

63. American Geriatrics Society Workgroup on Vitamin D Supplementation for Older Adults. Recommendations abstracted from the American Geriatrics Society consensus statement on vitamin D for prevention of falls and their consequences. J Am Geriatr Soc 2014;62(1):147–52.

64. de Jong MR, Van der Elst M, Hartholt KA. Drug-related falls in older patients: implicated drugs, consequences, and possible prevention strategies. Ther Adv Drug Saf 2013;4(4):147–54.

65. Haran MJ, Cameron ID, Ivers RQ, et al. Effect on falls of providing single lens distance vision glasses to multifocal glasses wearers: visible randomised controlled trial. BMJ 2010;340:c2265.

66. Frick KD, Kung JY, Parrish JM, et al. Evaluating the cost-effectiveness of fall prevention programs that reduce fall-related hip fractures in older adults. J Am Geriatr Soc 2010;58(1):136–41.

67. Spink MJ, Menz HB, Fotoohabadi MR, et al. Effectiveness of a multifaceted podiatry intervention to prevent falls in community dwelling older people with disabling foot pain: randomised controlled trial. BMJ 2011;342:d3411.

68. Gell NM, Patel KV. Rehabilitation services use of older adults according to fall-risk screening guidelines. J Am Geriatr Soc 2019;67(1):100–7.

69. Peterson EW, Clemson L. Understanding the role of occupational therapy in fall prevention for community-dwelling older adults. OT Practice 2008;13(3):CE1–8.

70. Burton E, Cavalheri V, Adams R, et al. Effectiveness of exercise programs to reduce falls in older people with dementia living in the community: a systematic review and meta-analysis. Clin Interv Aging 2015;10:421–34.

71. Lam FM, Huang MZ, Liao LR, et al. Physical exercise improves strength, balance, mobility, and endurance in people with cognitive impairment and dementia: a systematic review. J Physiother 2018;64(1):4–15.

72. Ohman H, Savikko N, Strandberg T, et al. Effects of exercise on functional performance and fall rate in subjects with mild or advanced Alzheimer's disease: secondary analyses of a randomized controlled study. Dement Geriatr Cogn Disord 2016;41(3–4):233–41.

73. Almeida SIL, Gomes da Silva M, Marques A. Home-based physical activity programs for people with dementia: systematic review and meta-analysis. Gerontologist 2019;gnz176. https://doi.org/10.1093/geront/gnz176.

74. Nyman SR, Ingram W, Sanders J, et al. Randomised controlled trial of the effect of Tai Chi on postural balance of people with dementia. Clin Interv Aging 2019;14: 2017–29.
75. Barrado-Martin Y, Heward M, Polman R, et al. Acceptability of a Dyadic Tai Chi intervention for older people living with dementia and their informal carers. J Aging Phys Act 2019;27(2):166–83.
76. Liu JYW, Kwan RYC, Lai CK, et al. A simplified 10-step Tai-chi programme to enable people with dementia to improve their motor performance: a feasibility study. Clin Rehabil 2018;32(12):1609–23.
77. Smith-Ray RL, Hughes SL, Prohaska TR, et al. Impact of cognitive training on balance and gait in older adults. J Gerontol B Psychol Sci Soc Sci 2015;70(3): 357–66.
78. Booth V, Hood V, Kearney F. Interventions incorporating physical and cognitive elements to reduce falls risk in cognitively impaired older adults: a systematic review. JBI Database System Rev Implement Rep 2016;14(5):110–35.
79. Scott I, Cooper C, Leverton M, et al. Effects of nonpharmacological interventions on functioning of people living with dementia at home: a systematic review of randomised controlled trials. Int J Geriatr Psychiatry 2019;34(10):1386–402.
80. Ries E. Improving the lives of people with dementia. PTinMotion 2018;14-24.
81. de Werd MM, Boelen D, Rikkert MG, et al. Errorless learning of everyday tasks in people with dementia. Clin Interv Aging 2013;8:1177–90.
82. Muir-Hunter SW, Montero-Odasso M. Gait cost of using a mobility aid in older adults with Alzheimer's disease. J Am Geriatr Soc 2016;64(2):437–8.
83. Bateni H, Maki BE. Assistive devices for balance and mobility: benefits, demands, and adverse consequences. Arch Phys Med Rehabil 2005;86(1):134–45.
84. Teri L, Logsdon RG, Uomoto J, et al. Behavioral treatment of depression in dementia patients: a controlled clinical trial. J Gerontol B Psychol Sci Soc Sci 1997;52(4):P159–66.
85. Teri L, Gibbons LE, McCurry SM, et al. Exercise plus behavioral management in patients with Alzheimer disease: a randomized controlled trial. JAMA 2003; 290(15):2015–22.
86. B.R.. Functional assessment staging (FAST). Psychopharmacol Bull 1988;24(4): 653–9.
87. Iaboni A, Van Ooteghem K, Marcil MN, et al. A palliative approach to falls in advanced dementia. Am J Geriatr Psychiatry 2018;26(4):407–15.
88. Biskup E, Vetter M, Wedding U. Fighting diagnostic and therapeutic nihilism in the elderly with cancer. Ann Palliat Med 2019. https://doi.org/10.21037/apm. 2019.08.03.
89. Naslund J. Visuospatial ability in relation to fall risk and dementia. Arch Neurol 2010;67(5):643.

Cognitive Impairment Evaluation and Management

Lauren McCollum, MD[a,b,*], Jason Karlawish, MD[b,c]

KEYWORDS

- Dementia • Mild cognitive impairment • Mental status examination
- Alzheimer's disease • Neuropsychiatric symptoms

KEY POINTS

- The goal of the diagnostic evaluation for cognitive impairment is to determine both the severity of impairment and the likely cause or causes.
- A knowledgeable informant is crucial for a reliable evaluation and, depending on the cause, patient care.
- The mental status examination should incorporate one or more validated instruments to assess cognition.
- An assessment of functional status informs both the diagnostic work-up and patient care.
- Environmental, psychological, and behavioral interventions are first line for neuropsychiatric symptoms and can be beneficial for cognition and function in cognitively impaired patients.

INTRODUCTION

Cognitive impairment is highly prevalent in the elderly and increases with advancing age.[1–3] Worldwide, dementia is estimated to affect 1.8% of people in their 60s, 5.1% of people in their 70s, 15.1% of people in their 80s, and 35.7% of people in their 90s.[3] A study from the Centers for Disease Control and Prevention using the 2011 Behavioral Risk Factor Surveillance survey found that 12.7% of respondents aged 60 years and older self-reported memory loss and confusion that had worsened in the preceding year.[4] Clinicians providing primary care to the elderly are often tasked with evaluating and managing cognitive concerns in their patient population.

[a] Penn Memory Center, University of Pennsylvania, Philadelphia, PA, USA; [b] Ralston House, Penn Memory Center, ATTN: Maria Crudele, 3615 Chestnut Street, Philadelphia, PA 19104-2612, USA; [c] Division of Geriatrics, Penn Memory Center, University of Pennsylvania, Philadelphia, PA, USA
* Corresponding author. Ralston House, Penn Memory Center, ATTN: Maria Crudele, 3615 Chestnut Street, Philadelphia, PA 19104-2612.
E-mail address: laurenmccollum@gmail.com
Twitter: @lauren_mccollum (L.M.); @jasonkarlawish (J.K.)

Med Clin N Am 104 (2020) 807–825
https://doi.org/10.1016/j.mcna.2020.06.007
0025-7125/20/© 2020 Elsevier Inc. All rights reserved.

medical.theclinics.com

APPROACH

To diagnose and treat a patient presenting with a cognitive complaint, the clinician uses a systematic approach that identifies the presence and severity of the impairment, the cognitive domains involved, the likely underlying causes, and the most appropriate interventions. Although some aspects of the work-up are completed for all patients (eg, selected laboratory tests and imaging), the decision to pursue a more detailed work-up is influenced by the goals of the evaluation. A brief discussion with the patient and family about the goal of the visit provides the necessary information to customize the approach.

The decision to refer a patient to a specialist can be considered at the close of the initial assessment. Cases of early-onset, rapidly progressive, or otherwise atypical cognitive impairment (eg, prominent language or social-behavioral symptoms with little or no memory loss) should be referred to a specialist.[5–7] Other factors that might influence a decision to refer include provider experience, clinic resources, patient preference, and availability of specialty centers.[2] One particularly compelling reason to refer to an academic center is interest in participation in clinical research.[2]

EVALUATION
History of Present Illness

A concern for cognitive change (commonly called a chief complaint of memory loss) triggers a work-up for cognitive impairment. This concern can be voiced by the patient or a knowledgeable informant. In general, a knowledgeable informant provides the most helpful historical information. The interview with the informant is best done privately, although this is not always practical or possible. Privacy allows the informant to feel comfortable describing the full extent of the problem. However, there is no need to hide this conversation from the patient. In our experience, patients are agreeable to allowing the informant to speak privately with the clinician if they are told that this is a routine part of the cognitive evaluation and they will have private time as well with the clinician.

The informant interview should begin with an assessment of how long the informant has known the patient and how frequently interaction with the patient occurs. An open-ended question about the reason for concern often provides a great deal of information. Next, it is helpful to take a step back and learn about the patient's cognitive achievements and background, including education, occupation, and living situation. The history covers all cognitive domains, including memory, attention, language, visuospatial processing, executive function, and social comportment, and addresses aspects of timing and tempo. Domains that are not covered when the informant answers an open-ended question can be addressed with a few key targeted questions (**Box 1**).

It is helpful to ask for examples that illustrate the patient's symptoms. These contextual details aid the physician in assessing the severity of the problem.

After establishing the pattern of cognitive impairment, the clinician should assess the functional impact of the symptoms. The activities of daily living are the instrumental activities of daily living (IADL), such as handling finances, cooking, managing medications, and using transportation, and the basic activities of daily living (BADL), which include bathing, dressing, grooming, feeding, and toileting.[8] An ecologically valid and holistic way to assess function is to begin by asking what a typical day is like or what the patient does to stay busy. The clinician should then ask questions to determine whether the patient's day-to-day activities represent a change from the baseline and, if so, are the result of cognitive problems. Questions should probe whether the

---

Box 1
Targeted questions to address cognitive domains

- Memory
  - Does the patient forget appointments or have difficulty keeping track of the day or time?
  - Does the patient repeat questions or comments?
  - Does the patient forget recent events or conversations?

- Attention
  - Does the patient have periods of decreased alertness?
  - Is the patient easily distracted?

- Language
  - Does the patient have word-finding difficulties? Struggle to find common words?
  - Does the patient have trouble communicating thoughts or understanding what is being said to them?

- Visuospatial processing
  - Does the patient tend to get lost or turned around?
  - Does the patient ever fail to see something that is right in front of them?

- Executive function
  - Can the patient successfully complete tasks that require multiple steps; for example, planning a trip or throwing a dinner party?
  - Can the patient use appliances and devices as well as they used to?

- Social comportment
  - Does the patient behave appropriately in social situations?
  - Has the patient become impulsive, careless, or unguarded?

Note: these questions refer to "the patient," but a more personal term, such as "your wife" or "your father," is used in practice.

---

patient is less efficient at performing tasks (ie, takes them longer) or makes errors and needs help.

Neuropsychiatric symptoms should be discussed, both because mood disorders, especially depression, can be a primary (and treatable) cause of cognitive change and because neurodegenerative diseases can cause various neuropsychiatric symptoms. For example, dementia with Lewy bodies (DLB) often results in anxiety, systematized delusions, and formed visual hallucinations.[9]

Sleep should be discussed, both because untreated sleep disorders (eg, obstructive sleep apnea [OSA]) may affect cognitive function in some older adults[10] and because neurodegenerative conditions are associated with sleep disturbance.[11,12] The possibility of rapid eye movement sleep behavior disorder (RBD), which is commonly seen in DLB, can be assessed for by asking whether the patient's arms and legs move during sleep, as if acting out dreams.[13]

A focused review of systems should inquire about gait dysfunction, falls, tremor, incontinence, and dysphagia. The past medical history should elucidate vascular risk factors and general medical, psychiatric, or neurologic diseases that could affect cognition. The social history assesses for illicit drug use, problematic alcohol use, and social stressors. The family history identifies genetic risk factors. In addition, the medication reconciliation should flag drugs that contribute to cognitive decline, particularly anticholinergic drugs.

The interview with the patient should include questions about cognitive symptoms and a typical day. This history from the patient is a part of the cognitive examination because it provides information about the patient's insight. Patients should be asked directly about their mood and hallucinations, because informants do not always know this very subjective information. Validated instruments for assessment of cognitive symptoms, functional decline, and neuropsychiatric features can augment the history of present illness and provide quantitative values that are helpful for both baseline and longitudinal assessments (**Table 1**).

Examination

The mental status examination should include both a "bedside" examination and the use of one or more validated instruments to assess cognition and, if applicable, mood (**Table 1**). There are some scenarios in which the results of formal cognitive tests must be interpreted with caution. For example, the psychometric test performance of persons with limited education, particularly less than high school, and for whom English is a second language may underestimate their cognitive abilities. In addition, certain cognitive deficits, such as marked impairments in language or attention, can cause performance on tests that is markedly poorer than expected.

The bedside mental status examination touches on the various cognitive domains. From the start of the encounter with the patient, the clinician makes observations regarding the patient's cognition and behavior. While taking the history, the clinician is also taking note of the patient's affect, social comportment, speech, facial expressions, and insight. The versions of the bedside mental status examination are limitless, and clinicians often tailor the examination based on preference, patient factors, and the evolving differential diagnosis. The various bedside tests available are best organized according to the cognitive domains they test (**Box 2**).

Next, the clinician should perform a focused neurologic examination designed to detect findings that the chief complaint and history suggest might be present (**Box 3**).

A brief general medical examination with attention to the cardiac and pulmonary systems assesses for signs of a non-neurologic problems that could affect cognition.

Referral for a formal neuropsychological evaluation should be considered when there is significant psychiatric comorbidity or when there is a mismatch between the history and the cognitive test results—for example, a patient whose cognitive test performance is normal but in whom a decline from baseline is still suspected. More in-depth testing may reveal deficits too subtle to show up on simpler office-based tests. Neuropsychologists can also assist in refining the differential diagnosis by identifying patterns of cognitive dysfunction.

Determining Level of Impairment

The history and examination provide clinicians with the data needed to characterize the level of impairment:

- *Subjective cognitive decline (SCD)* describes patients who have expressed concern for cognitive change but perform normally on cognitive testing.[14]
- *Mild cognitive impairment (MCI)* describes patients with concern for cognitive change, voiced by the patient or the informant; objective evidence of impaired cognition in one or more cognitive domains; and relative preservation of independent function, such that the patient does not meet criteria for dementia. Typically, a person with MCI is less efficient in performing IADLs.[15] MCI can be staged as early or late, depending on the severity of symptoms.
- *Dementia* describes a patient with concern for cognitive decline, objective cognitive impairment, and disability. Dementia is distinguished from MCI in that the cognitive symptoms of dementia are severe enough to interfere with performance of day-to-day activities.[16] Dementia can be further characterized as mild, moderate, or severe, based on functional status. In mild-stage dementia,

Table 1
Selected validated instruments for assessment of cognition, functional status, and neuropsychiatric symptoms

Instrument	Description	How It Is Administered	Scoring	Considerations
Functional Activities Questionnaire	Informant questionnaire about patient's performance of day-to-day tasks	Examiner administers to informant	Score range: 0–30; lower scores c/w less impairment; ≥9, impaired function and possible cognitive impairment	• Takes 5 min • Must have reliable informant • May help identify safety concerns and areas of need
General Practitioner Assessment of Cognition	Psychometric test of memory, language, executive function, and structured informant interview	Examiner administers psychometric test to patient and interviews informant	Patient examination (out of 9): 0–4, cognitive impairment; 5–8, need more information (interview informant); 9, normal. Informant interview (out of 6): 0–3, cognitive impairment	• Takes 4–5 min • >80% sensitivity and specificity
GDS	30 yes/no questions about depressive symptoms; 15-item version also available (GDS-15)	Examiner administers to patient, or patient self-administers	Score range (full version): 0–30; ≥14, increased depressive symptoms; 11–13, borderline	• May be less reliable for more impaired patients
IQCODE	26-item informant questionnaire with 5-point Likert scale; shorter 16-item version (Short IQCODE) also available	Informant self-administers	Score range 1–5 (mean Likert score); higher scores c/w more impairment	• 75%–87.6% sensitive and 65%–91% specific for dementia • 71.1%–82.6% sensitive and 69.0%–83.0% specific for MCI • Unknown optimal cut points
Memory Impairment Screen	Brief psychometric delayed and cued recall test	Examiner administers to patient	Score range: 0–8; ≤4, possible cognitive impairment	• Takes 4 min • 43%–86% sensitive and 93%–97% specific for dementia • Works for visually impaired (no writing or drawing component)

(continued on next page)

Table 1
(continued)

Instrument	Description	How It Is Administered	Scoring	Considerations
Mini-Cog	Psychometric test of memory, executive function, language, and praxis using clock draw and 3-word recall test	Examiner administers to patient	Score range 0–5; higher score c/w less cognitive impairment	• Takes 3–4 min • 76%–100% sensitive and 54%–85.2% specific for dementia • Low sensitivity for MCI • May perform better in low-education populations
Mini Mental State Examination	Psychometric test of memory, attention, orientation, language, and praxis	Examiner administers to patient	Score range: 0–30; 21–24, mild dementia; 13–20, moderate dementia; 3-point change considered clinically significant	• Takes 7–10 min • 88.3% sensitive and 86.2% specific for dementia with a cut point of 23/24 or 24/25 • Limited sensitivity and specificity for MCI • Has copyright restrictions
Montreal Cognitive Assessment	Psychometric test of memory, executive function, language, and praxis; designed to detect MCI	Examiner administers to patient	Score range 0–30; higher score c/w less cognitive impairment	• Takes 10 min • 80%–100% sensitive and 50%–76% specific for MCI using cut point of 25/26
NPI-Q	Informant questionnaire on 12 behavioral symptoms (items are yes/no; yes answers get 1–3 severity rating) and caregiver distress (1–5)	Informant self-administers	NPI-Q severity score range: 0–36. NPI-Q distress score: 0–60; higher scores c/w more severe behavioral symptoms and caregiver distress	• Takes 5 min • Must have reliable informant • Assesses for behavioral symptoms associated with multiple dementia syndromes

See the text for definitions of MCI and dementia.

Abbreviations: c/w, consistent with; GDS, Geriatric Depression Scale; IQCODE, Informant Questionnaire on Cognitive Decline in the Elderly; MCI, mild cognitive impairment; NPI-Q, Neuropsychiatric Inventory Questionnaire.

Data from Lin, J. S., et al. Screening for cognitive impairment in older adults: A systematic review for the U.S. Preventive Services Task Force. *Ann Intern Med.* 2013 **159**(9): 601-612.

Box 2

Selected components of a bedside mental status examination grouped by cognitive domain

- Orientation
  - State name, month, date, year, day of the week, season, and current location

- Attention
  - Spell "world" forward and backward
  - State months of the year in reverse order
  - Count backward from 100 by 7s

- Memory
  - Repeat 3 words and remember them for 5 minutes
  - Describe what has been going on in the news lately

- Language
  - Name 3 common items (eg, thumb, knuckles, collar, pointed to by the examiner)
  - Repeat a phrase (eg, "Traffic conditions are expected to be heavy today.")
  - Provide a speech sample (eg, by describing a picture or current event)

- Visuospatial processing
  - Draw a clock (also tests executive function)
  - Bisect a line

- Executive function
  - Name as many words that begin with the letter F as you can think of in 1 minute
  - State the letters of the alphabet, alternating with sequential numbers (ie, "A1B2" and so on)

Box 3

Focused neurologic examination for a patient with a cognitive complaint

- Cranial nerves:
  - Assess for masked facies or reduced eye blink rate
  - Listen for dysarthria
  - Look for facial asymmetry, including flattening of the nasolabial fold
  - Determine whether eye movements and visual fields are full

- Motor, sensory, and reflexes
  - Test briefly, assessing for focal weakness, fasciculations, or hyperreflexia concerning for amyotrophic lateral sclerosis, which is sometimes comorbid with frontotemporal dementia, or other asymmetry suggestive of a focal lesion (eg, stroke, tumor)

- Tone
  - Assess for cogwheel rigidity at the elbows, wrists, and neck by asking the patients to relax and allow you to move their bodies for them

- Coordination and extrapyramidal function
  - Evaluate rapid alternating movements (eg, by having the patients alternate striking their thighs with a closed fist and open palm)
  - Evaluate for emergence of a rest tremor by having the patients rest their hands in their laps and count backward from 20 to zero with eyes closed

- Gait and postural stability
  - Have patients stand without the use of their hands
  - Observe gait (noting arm swing, posture, stride length, and turn)
  - Assess tandem gait
  - Use pull test to assess for postural instability

the patient is independent in BADL and requires some assistance with IADL. In the moderate stage, the patient requires some assistance with BADL and requires assistance with or is dependent in IADL. In the severe stage, the patient requires assistance with or is dependent in BADL and is dependent in IADL.

The labels MCI and dementia both denote a concern that a disease, most likely a brain disease, is causing the cognitive problems, and so should not be applied if the deficits are explained by delirium or some other cause that is not a brain disease, such as decompensated congestive heart failure.

Work-up

Patients with cognitive impairment should be screened for hypothyroidism and vitamin B_{12} deficiency, because these entities can cause cognitive decline that may improve with treatment.[17–19] It is reasonable to obtain a complete blood count with differential and comprehensive metabolic panel to screen for other general medical problems (eg, anemia, kidney or liver failure, electrolyte derangements) that could affect cognition.[17,20] Depending on clinical context, clinicians may consider ordering other laboratory tests, such as folate, vitamin D, heavy metal screen, erythrocyte sedimentation rate, C-reactive protein, antinuclear antibodies, Lyme serologies, human immunodeficiency virus-1/2 immunoassay, and rapid plasma reagin.[16,20,21] Patients in whom OSA is suspected should undergo a sleep study or be referred to a sleep specialist.

All patients with cognitive impairment should undergo structural brain imaging. Brain imaging is not indicated in patients with SCD because normal age-related changes can overlap with the early atrophic changes seen in neurodegenerative disease.[22] Thus, structural brain imaging, in the absence of objective cognitive impairment, is often clinically uninterpretable, because mild atrophy could be age related, and a normal result does not rule out the small possibility of occult disorder.

Although both computed tomography (CT) and magnetic resonance imaging (MRI) are acceptable, the preferred brain imaging modality for cognitive impairment is MRI without contrast, which has greater diagnostic yield and avoids ionizing radiation. CT without contrast, which is generally less costly, is a suitable alternative when MRI is contraindicated or otherwise unable to be obtained.[16] Imaging enables the clinician both to assess for unexpected structural findings that could be affecting cognition (eg, a tumor, silent stroke, or subdural hematoma) and to identify features suggestive of specific underlying neurologic diagnoses.[23] Several of the diseases that cause dementia have characteristic imaging findings (eg, hippocampal and posterior parietal atrophy in Alzheimer disease [AD]) (**Table 2**).[24] However, these findings can be subtle, and the relationship between imaging findings and underlying disorder is best thought of as probabilistic, with the most compelling cases being those in which the clinical symptoms and the imaging findings align.

MRI is also helpful for identifying cerebrovascular disease, because many types of vascular brain injuries have identifiable imaging correlates. White matter hyperintensities, which are suggestive of chronic small vessel ischemic disease, are commonly related to typical cardiovascular risk factors (eg, hypertension, smoking),[25,26] but are also commonly seen in AD.[27,28] Similarly, cerebral microbleeds (CMBs) are commonly seen in both vascular cognitive impairment and AD. Deep subcortical CMBs are usually hypertensive in origin, whereas lobar CMBs are more often associated with cerebral amyloid, and thus are suggestive of AD.[29]

Normal-pressure hydrocephalus (NPH) can be suggested, but not definitively diagnosed, by characteristic imaging findings, including ventriculomegaly and disproportionately enlarged subarachnoid space.[30] There has been growing recognition that

Table 2	
Common MRI findings in selected causes of progressive cognitive impairment	
Neurologic Disease	**Common MRI Findings**
AD	Atrophy affecting the hippocampi, MTLs, and posterior parietal lobes[a]
DLB	Normal MRI or mild, nonspecific atrophy with relative sparing of MTLs[b]
Frontotemporal dementia	Atrophy of frontal and temporal lobes[c]
Vascular cognitive impairment	Multiple bilateral chronic lacunar strokes; white matter hyperintensities[c]
Normal-pressure hydrocephalus	Ventriculomegaly; disproportionately enlarged subarachnoid space[d]

Abbreviation: MTLs, medial temporal lobes.
[a] *Data from* Whitwell, J. L. Progression of atrophy in Alzheimer disease and related disorders. *Neurotox Res.* 2010 **18**(3-4): 339-346.
[b] *Data from* Yousaf, T., et al. Neuroimaging in Lewy body dementia. *J Neurol.* 2019 **266**(1): 1-26.
[c] *Data from* Masdeu, J. C. Neuroimaging of Diseases Causing Dementia. *Neurol Clin.* 2020 **38**(1): 65-94.
[d] *Data from* Graff-Radford, N. R. and D. T. Jones. Normal Pressure Hydrocephalus. *Continuum (Minneap Minn).* 2019 **25**(1): 165-186.

mixed dementia (ie, multiple disorders together causing the impairment) is common, particularly in the elderly.[31,32]

If the diagnosis is still unclear, additional studies or a referral to a cognitive specialist may be needed. A fluorodeoxyglucose-PET scan of the brain can distinguish between frontotemporal dementia (FTD) and AD. Amyloid PET scans are approved for the detection of amyloid by the Food and Drug Administration (FDA) in the United States, but, as of this writing, are not covered by any insurance plans. Cerebral spinal fluid from a lumbar puncture (LP) can be tested for biomarkers of specific diseases, including AD (with amyloid-beta-42 and phosphorylated tau),[33] sporadic Creutzfeldt-Jakob disease (with real-time quaking-induced conversion),[34,35] autoimmune and paraneoplastic encephalitides (with respective panels),[36] and other inflammatory entities (with protein and white blood cell counts).[37] A high-volume LP, preceded and followed by cognitive and timed walking tests, can evaluate for NPH, in the appropriate context of the clinical triad (gait disturbance, urinary incontinence, and dementia) and suggestive neuroimaging.[30]

Providing a Diagnosis

Discussions about the diagnosis should include information about the level of impairment (MCI or dementia) and the causes. If the patient has SCD, the clinician should explain that cognitive testing was normal and provide prognostic information. Individuals with SCD are at a modestly increased risk of progression to MCI and dementia over subsequent years, compared with the general population.[38–40] It is reasonable to follow the patient over time with repeated cognitive assessments to assess for onset of objective cognitive decline. Education about cognitive aging is warranted as well.

Clinicians giving a diagnosis of MCI discuss with patients and their families the meaning of the diagnosis and its prognosis.[2] People with MCI can progress to dementia, remain in an MCI state, or revert to normal cognition, and studies have shown that all 3 outcomes are common.[2] Each year, 5% to 20% of patients with MCI progress to dementia.[20]

A diagnosis of dementia merits disclosure of the disease that is causing it, or, if that cause is uncertain, an offer for referral to a specialist. **Table 3** lists abbreviated diagnostic criteria of selected commonly diagnosed neurodegenerative diseases that cause dementia. Some common dementia syndromes, such as NPH and vascular dementia, do not have a single set of widely agreed-on diagnostic criteria.

If the patient has a neurodegenerative disease, it is important to stage the disease. Diagnostic disclosure should explain that these conditions are gradually progressive, and the goal of any intervention is to slow down or stabilize the functional decline and other symptoms. Family members in particular need to understand this so they can

Table 3	
Abbreviated diagnostic criteria for commonly diagnosed neurodegenerative dementias	
Diagnosis	**Abbreviated Diagnostic Criteria**
AD dementia[a]	• Progressive, insidious decline with dementia-level impairment • Amnestic or nonamnestic presentation ○ Amnestic (most common): impairment in learning and episodic memory ○ Nonamnestic: language (particularly word finding), visuospatial, or executive function • Not better explained by another entity • Can increase certainty with imaging or CSF biomarkers
Behavioral variant frontotemporal dementia[b]	• Progressive cognitive and/or behavioral decline • Need 3 of the following: ○ Behavioral disinhibition ○ Apathy or inertia ○ Compulsive, ritualistic, or perseverative behavior ○ Hyperorality ○ Dysexecutive presentation with relative sparing of memory and visuospatial function • Can increase certainty with imaging biomarkers
DLB[c]	• Progressive cognitive decline with dementia-level impairment • Core clinical features: ○ Fluctuating cognition ○ Well-formed visual hallucinations ○ RBD ○ Parkinsonism • Supportive features: sensitivity to antipsychotics, postural instability, falls, dysautonomia, delusions, anxiety, apathy, depression • Probable DLB: 2 core features or 1 core feature plus 1 indicative biomarker • Possible DLB: 1 core feature or 1 indicative biomarker

Abbreviation: CSF, cerebrospinal fluid.

[a] *Data from* McKhann, G. M., Knopman D.S., Chertkow H., et al. The diagnosis of dementia due to Alzheimer's disease: recommendations from the National Institute on Aging-Alzheimer's Association workgroups on diagnostic guidelines for Alzheimer's disease. *Alzheimers Dement.* 2011 7(3): 263-269.

[b] *Data from* Rascovsky K., Hodges J.R., Knopman D., et al. Sensitivity of revised diagnostic criteria for the behavioural variant of frontotemporal dementia. *Brain.* 2011 **134**(Pt 9): 2456-2477.

[c] *Data from* McKeith I. G., Boeve B.F., Dickson D.W., et al. Diagnosis and management of dementia with Lewy bodies: Fourth consensus report of the DLB Consortium. *Neurology.* 2017 **89**(1): 88-100.

help the patient live well with the disease and prepare for the future. Each cause of dementia has its own prognosis, but clinicians should emphasize that there is variability in rates of progression.

TREATMENT OF COGNITIVE IMPAIRMENT

If the work-up uncovers an alternative cause of cognitive impairment (eg, hypothyroidism, OSA), it should be treated. Vascular contributors to cognitive decline, such as hypertension, diabetes, and smoking, should be addressed. Medications that contribute to cognitive impairment, particularly anticholinergic medications, should be tapered or stopped, if possible.[2] NPH is treated with ventriculoperitoneal shunting.

Pharmacotherapy

As of 2020, there are no approved therapies shown to modify neurodegenerative disorders, although many are being studied in clinical trials. The available medications are symptomatic treatments.

Acetylcholinesterase inhibitors

Acetylcholinesterase inhibitors, including donepezil, galantamine, and rivastigmine, are labeled for use in AD dementia and may also be effective for vascular dementia and DLB.[41] Acetylcholinesterase inhibitors can worsen behaviors in FTD,[42] and there is insufficient evidence of efficacy in MCI.[2] The goal of treatment with acetylcholinesterase inhibitors is to improve or stabilize memory and attention by inhibiting the breakdown of acetylcholine, a neurotransmitter released by cholinergic neurons in the basal forebrain, an area known to be affected by AD.[43] Common side effects include diarrhea, nausea, leg cramps, abnormal dreams, and bradycardia. Patients with a history of bradycardia or conduction abnormalities should not be prescribed acetylcholinesterase inhibitors. Some patients who cannot tolerate oral donepezil because of gastrointestinal side effects are able to tolerate the rivastigmine patch.[41] If the side effects persist and are bothersome, the clinician should consider discontinuing the medication because any mild symptomatic benefit is likely to be overshadowed by side effects. Patients and families should be advised that, because the benefits of acetylcholinesterase inhibitors tend to be subtle, it is often not obvious that the medication is helping, even in patients who are doing a little better than they otherwise would be.

Memantine

Memantine, an N-methyl-D-aspartate (NMDA) receptor antagonist, is thought to work by blocking the effects of excess glutamate and by upregulating NMDA receptor expression.[44] Memantine is indicated for use in moderate to severe AD,[45] and there is also evidence to support off-label use in mild to moderate vascular dementia.[46] Memantine has been shown to confer modest improvements in thinking, everyday functioning, behavior and mood.[47] Although memantine is generally well tolerated, the most common side effect is dizziness.[47] As is the case with acetylcholinesterase inhibitors, patients and families should be counseled that the benefits of memantine tend to be subtle.

A common practice for patients with AD, vascular dementia, or mixed dementia is to start an acetylcholinesterase inhibitor at the mild dementia stage and to add memantine to the drug regimen when the patient progresses to a moderate stage of dementia.

Environmental, Psychological, and Behavioral Interventions

Various lifestyle interventions, which can both improve quality of life and slow functional decline, are paramount in the management of cognitive impairment. When giving a dementia diagnosis, clinicians should counsel patients and families to work to create a safe, structured, social, and engaged day. All patients with SCD, MCI, and dementia should be active physically, mentally, and socially. Activities that combine physical, mental, and social activity in some way are especially valuable; for example, joining a book club (which is mentally and socially stimulating) or taking a dance class (which is stimulating in all 3 regards). Unfortunately, the Covid-19 pandemic has rendered many common lifestyle measures unsafe for elderly individuals because of infection risk in group settings. Caregivers should endeavor to facilitate stimulating experiences that are also safe; for example, home exercise programs and video conference–based social experiences.

Exercise
In people with dementia, exercise programs have been shown to improve or stabilize functional status[48] and cognition.[49] The type and amount of exercise with the best evidence basis in people with MCI or AD is 3 or 4 ~45-minute moderate-intensity aerobic exercise workouts per week.[49] Mind-body exercises (eg, yoga, tai chi) have also been shown to improve cognition in MCI.[50]

Cognitive stimulation
Studies have shown some benefit to cognitively stimulating activities, including computer activities, video games, and virtual reality programs for MCI[51] and dementia.[52,53] It is reasonable to refer patients to cognitive fitness/rehabilitation programs to the extent that they are available and affordable. Clinicians should also encourage pursuit of cognitively stimulating activities in day-to-day life. The choice of activity depends on the abilities and interests of the patient. Mindfulness meditation may help patients with MCI build cognitive reserve, become more socially engaged, and feel better about their diagnoses.[54] Speech therapy can be helpful for people with prominent language disturbance.

Social engagement
Poor social engagement (ie, loneliness) is associated with an increased risk of dementia,[55,56] and community cultural engagement (eg, visiting museums, going to the theater) may be a protective factor for dementia risk.[57] Social engagement is most stimulating when it involves people outside the patient's innermost circle. Some caregivers try to provide round-the-clock care and companionship, but it is in the best interest of both patients and caregivers to intersperse interactions with other people, which can take the form of visiting aides, an adult day program, or having an old friend take the patient out for lunch once a week.

Nutrition
The Mediterranean diet has been associated with a lower risk of conversion from MCI to dementia.[58,59] Patients with dementia are at increased risk of malnutrition, and nutritional status may have some bearing on functional status.[60] For patients at risk for malnutrition, caregivers should provide routine meals and snacks. (Often, even if they say they are not hungry, they will eat once a meal is served to them.) Nutrition supplements, such as shakes, can provide additional nutrition.[61] Patients should avoid moderate or heavy alcohol use.

Sleep
Behavioral interventions for sleep disturbance include counseling about sleep hygiene, light therapy, and referral for cognitive behavioral therapy for insomnia.[62,63] Sleep disturbance can be exacerbated by excessive napping and insufficient daytime

activity. Crafting a more active day that involves leaving the house during daylight hours can result in improved sleep.

MANAGEMENT OF NEUROPSYCHIATRIC SYMPTOMS

Neuropsychiatric symptoms are common in people with cognitive impairment. Depression can itself cause cognitive impairment (pseudodementia), which can improve with appropriate treatment.[64] Depressive symptoms are also a common neuropsychiatric manifestation of dementing disorders, as are anxiety, irritability, agitation, apathy, hallucinations, and delusions. Although it is common for patients to require pharmacologic interventions, nonpharmacologic strategies (ie, behavioral interventions, environmental modifications, and lifestyle changes) are first line for management of dementia-related neuropsychiatric symptoms.

Nonpharmacologic Management of Neuropsychiatric Symptoms

Nonpharmacologic strategies for management of neuropsychiatric symptoms should always be considered first line instead of pharmacologic treatments, especially antipsychotic medications. Assessment for underlying causes of neuropsychiatric symptoms should be the first step. Issues such as pain, fatigue, or problems with the environment (eg, temperature, lighting) should be addressed. Environmental adaptations can range from raising the shades during the day; to building a soothing multisensory environment with music, art, plants, and aromatherapy[65]; to relocating the patient to a memory care facility. Interventions designed to equip family caregivers with strategies to manage neuropsychiatric symptoms have the best evidence basis.[66] Caregivers should be encouraged to seek out caregiving workshops, support groups, and other resources. Caregiver training can teach cognitive reframing, stress reduction techniques, and other skills for addressing neuropsychiatric symptoms in ways that are personalized to the needs of individual patients.

Pharmacologic Treatment of Neuropsychiatric Symptoms

Selective serotonin reuptake inhibitors (SSRIs) are often used for treatment of depression and anxiety in dementia, despite a weak evidence basis for this practice.[67,68] Nevertheless, because SSRIs are first line for late-life depression,[69] it is reasonable to treat dementia-related depression and anxiety with SSRIs.[41] The SSRIs most commonly used in this population are sertraline, citalopram, and escitalopram.[69] SSRIs are also used to treat dementia-related agitation and psychosis, often in an effort to avoid the notable side effects of antipsychotics. The SSRI with the most solid evidence basis for this practice is citalopram.[67,70] Our practice is to start with sertraline, because it is associated with a lower risk of QT prolongation than citalopram or escitalopram.[71]

Antidepressants with other mechanisms of action (eg, duloxetine, bupropion, mirtazapine, trazodone) are also sometimes used to target dementia-related mood symptoms in tandem with some other symptom (eg, targeting neuropathic pain and depression with duloxetine, or low appetite and anxiety with mirtazapine). Tricyclic antidepressants are often avoided because of their anticholinergic side effects.[41] Buspirone, which is labeled to treat generalized anxiety disorder, can be used to manage anxiety in this population, and there is weak evidence to suggest that it could be helpful in managing dementia-related agitation.[72,73] Benzodiazepines should be avoided. They increase the risk of falls, worsen cognition, and soon lead to dependence.

Atypical antipsychotic drugs, such as quetiapine, olanzapine, risperidone, and pimavanserin, are often used to treat dementia-related agitation and psychosis, despite an FDA warning of increased mortality.[74] Because of the risks, it is imperative that nonpharmacologic interventions be tried before initiating treatment with antipsychotics.[75] Hallucinations and delusions should only be treated pharmacologically to the extent that they are distressing to the patient or disruptive for care or safety. Clinicians should advise patients and their families about the risks and plan to withdraw the drug if there is no response in 4 weeks and, if there is a response, to attempt to wean the drug within 4 months.[75] Pimavanserin is labeled for treatment of Parkinson disease psychosis, and there is evidence to support its use in dementia-related psychosis.[76]

Sleep disturbances are common in cognitive disorders.[77] If nonpharmacologic strategies fail, there are several medication options. Despite studies indicating a lack of efficacy, melatonin is commonly used for insomnia in people with dementia because of its good safety profile.[78] Trazodone may be an effective and reasonably safe treatment of dementia-related sleep disturbance.[78]

CONSIDERATIONS

Safety is a major issue for patients with cognitive impairment. Clinicians should be prepared to discuss driving with patients and families. Some patients with MCI and mild dementia can drive safely, whereas others cannot. People with moderate or severe dementia should not drive. Some states mandate that clinicians formally report unsafe drivers. When in doubt, a driver evaluation, performed at a rehabilitation center by an occupational therapist, can clarify whether the patient is safe behind the wheel.

Varying levels of supervision are needed for patients with cognitive disorders. Many patients with MCI or mild dementia need little supervision except in error-prone domains, particularly managing finances and medications. Patients with moderate to severe dementia should have near-constant supervision. Potential hazards for cognitively impaired patients should be addressed proactively; for example, removing guns from the home and turning off the gas to the stove. Gait instability during the examination or report of falls warrants referral to physical therapy to aid in fall prevention. Patients with dysphagia should see a speech pathologist.

Patients with cognitive impairment should be advised, together with their families, to plan for the future, which could include discussions about advance directives, powers of attorney, finances, and living arrangements.[2]

CLINICS CARE POINTS

- A knowledgeable informant is a crucial source of important historical information.
- Ensure cognitive impairment is objectively present before ordering a work-up. Structural neuroimaging is not indicated in patients with subjective decline only.
- The standard of care for MCI is lifestyle interventions. If prescribing a medication for MCI (eg, donepezil), patients must be counseled that the treatment is off label.
- Behavioral interventions are first line for neuropsychiatric symptoms of dementia. Interventions designed to educate and support caregivers are particularly effective.

SUMMARY

In conclusion, clinicians should take a systematic approach to evaluating and managing patients with cognitive impairment. A careful history, with input from a knowledgeable informant, often provides the most salient information. The patient's cognitive testing, examination, imaging, and laboratory results help complete the picture. The diagnosis consists of 2 parts: a level of impairment (eg, MCI or dementia) and probable cause (eg, AD, DLB, vascular dementia). Patients with unusual presentations or who are interested in research should be referred to an academic memory or cognitive center. Regardless of the underlying disorder, treatment is symptomatic, and nonpharmacologic interventions are preferred to pharmacologic ones for neuropsychiatric symptoms. Safety is a "moving target" in patients with cognitive impairment and should be a focus for clinicians.

DISCLOSURE

The authors have nothing to disclose.

REFERENCES

1. Hu C, Yu D, Sun X, et al. The prevalence and progression of mild cognitive impairment among clinic and community populations: a systematic review and meta-analysis. Int Psychogeriatr 2017;29(10):1595–608.
2. Petersen RC, Lopez O, Armstrong MJ, et al. Practice guideline update summary: mild cognitive impairment: report of the guideline development, dissemination, and implementation Subcommittee of the American Academy of Neurology. Neurology 2018;90(3):126–35.
3. Cao Q, Tan CC, Xu W, et al. The prevalence of dementia: a systematic review and meta-analysis. J Alzheimers Dis 2020;73(3):1157–66.
4. Centers for Disease Control and Prevention. Self-reported increased confusion or memory loss and associated functional difficulties among adults aged >/= 60 years - 21 States, 2011. MMWR Morb Mortal Wkly Rep 2013;62(18):347–50.
5. Shinagawa S, Catindig JA, Block NR, et al. When a little knowledge can be dangerous: false-positive diagnosis of behavioral variant frontotemporal dementia among community clinicians. Dement Geriatr Cogn Disord 2016;41(1-2):99–108.
6. Santacruz KS, Swagerty D. Early diagnosis of dementia. Am Fam Physician 2001;63(4):703–13, 717–8.
7. Hugo J, Ganguli M. Dementia and cognitive impairment: epidemiology, diagnosis, and treatment. Clin Geriatr Med 2014;30(3):421–42.
8. Lawton MP, Brody EM. Assessment of older people: self-maintaining and instrumental activities of daily living. Gerontologist 1969;9(3):179–86.
9. Del Ser T, McKeith I, Anand R, et al. Dementia with lewy bodies: findings from an international multicentre study. Int J Geriatr Psychiatry 2000;15(11):1034–45.
10. Cross N, Lampit A, Pye J, et al. Is obstructive sleep apnoea related to neuropsychological function in healthy older adults? a systematic review and meta-analysis. Neuropsychol Rev 2017;27(4):389–402.
11. Ju YE, Lucey BP, Holtzman DM. Sleep and alzheimer disease pathology–a bidirectional relationship. Nat Rev Neurol 2014;10(2):115–9.
12. Yaffe K, Laffan AM, Harrison SL, et al. Sleep-disordered breathing, hypoxia, and risk of mild cognitive impairment and dementia in older women. JAMA 2011;306(6):613–9.
13. McKeith IG, Boeve BF, Dickson DW, et al. Diagnosis and management of dementia with Lewy bodies: Fourth consensus report of the DLB Consortium. Neurology 2017;89(1):88–100.
14. Jessen F, Amariglio RE, van Boxtel M, et al. A conceptual framework for research on subjective cognitive decline in preclinical Alzheimer's disease. Alzheimers Dement 2014;10(6):844–52.

15. Petersen RC. Mild Cognitive Impairment. Continuum (Minneap Minn) 2016;22(2 Dementia):404–18.
16. Gale SA, Acar D, Daffner KR. Dementia. Am J Med 2018;131(10):1161–9.
17. Knopman DS, DeKosky ST, Cummings JL, et al. Practice parameter: diagnosis of dementia (an evidence-based review). Report of the Quality Standards Subcommittee of the American Academy of Neurology. Neurology 2001;56(9):1143–53.
18. Dugbartey AT. Neurocognitive aspects of hypothyroidism. Arch Intern Med 1998; 158(13):1413–8.
19. Eastley R, Wilcock GK, Bucks RS. Vitamin B12 deficiency in dementia and cognitive impairment: the effects of treatment on neuropsychological function. Int J Geriatr Psychiatry 2000;15(3):226–33.
20. Langa KM, Levine DA. The diagnosis and management of mild cognitive impairment: a clinical review. JAMA 2014;312(23):2551–61.
21. Arvanitakis Z, Shah RC, Bennett DA. Diagnosis and management of dementia: review. JAMA 2019;322(16):1589–99.
22. Bakkour A, Morris JC, Wolk DA, et al. The effects of aging and Alzheimer's disease on cerebral cortical anatomy: specificity and differential relationships with cognition. Neuroimage 2013;76:332–44.
23. Staffaroni AM, Elahi FM, McDermott D, et al. Neuroimaging in dementia. Semin Neurol 2017;37(5):510–37.
24. Whitwell JL. Progression of atrophy in Alzheimer's disease and related disorders. Neurotox Res 2010;18(3-4):339–46.
25. Abraham HM, Wolfson L, Moscufo N, et al. Cardiovascular risk factors and small vessel disease of the brain: Blood pressure, white matter lesions, and functional decline in older persons. J Cereb Blood Flow Metab 2016;36(1):132–42.
26. Longstreth WT Jr, Arnold AM, Beauchamp NJ Jr, et al. Incidence, manifestations, and predictors of worsening white matter on serial cranial magnetic resonance imaging in the elderly: the Cardiovascular Health Study. Stroke 2005;36(1):56–61.
27. Alosco ML, Sugarman MA, Besser LM, et al. A clinicopathological investigation of white matter hyperintensities and alzheimer's disease neuropathology. J Alzheimers Dis 2018;63(4):1347–60.
28. Damulina A, Pirpamer L, Seiler S, et al. White matter hyperintensities in alzheimer's disease: a lesion probability mapping study. J Alzheimers Dis 2019; 68(2):789–96.
29. Graff-Radford J, Simino J, Kantarci K, et al. Neuroimaging correlates of cerebral microbleeds: the ARIC Study (Atherosclerosis Risk in Communities). Stroke 2017; 48(11):2964–72.
30. Graff-Radford NR, Jones DT. Normal pressure hydrocephalus. Continuum (Minneap Minn) 2019;25(1):165–86.
31. James BD, Wilson RS, Boyle PA, et al. TDP-43 stage, mixed pathologies, and clinical Alzheimer's-type dementia. Brain 2016;139(11):2983–93.
32. Yu L, Boyle PA, Leurgans S, et al. Effect of common neuropathologies on progression of late life cognitive impairment. Neurobiol Aging 2015;36(7):2225–31.
33. Olsson B, Lautner R, Andreasson U, et al. CSF and blood biomarkers for the diagnosis of Alzheimer's disease: a systematic review and meta-analysis. Lancet Neurol 2016;15(7):673–84.
34. Hermann P, Laux M, Glatzel M, et al. Validation and utilization of amended diagnostic criteria in Creutzfeldt-Jakob disease surveillance. Neurology 2018;91(4): e331–8.
35. Fiorini M, Iselle G, Perra D, et al. High diagnostic accuracy of RT-QuIC assay in a prospective study of patients with suspected sCJD. Int J Mol Sci 2020;21(3):880.

36. Wesley SF, Ferguson D. Autoimmune encephalitides and rapidly progressive dementias. Semin Neurol 2019;39(2):283–92.
37. Geschwind MD. Rapidly progressive dementia. Continuum (Minneap Minn) 2016; 22(2 Dementia):510–37.
38. Reisberg B, Shulman MB, Torossian C, et al. Outcome over seven years of healthy adults with and without subjective cognitive impairment. Alzheimers Dement 2010;6(1):11–24.
39. Fernandez-Blazquez MA, Avila-Villanueva M, Maestu F, et al. Specific features of subjective cognitive decline predict faster conversion to mild cognitive impairment. J Alzheimers Dis 2016;52(1):271–81.
40. Mitchell AJ, Beaumont H, Ferguson D, et al. Risk of dementia and mild cognitive impairment in older people with subjective memory complaints: meta-analysis. Acta Psychiatr Scand 2014;130(6):439–51.
41. Tisher A, Salardini A. A comprehensive update on treatment of dementia. Semin Neurol 2019;39(2):167–78.
42. Mendez MF, Shapira JS, McMurtray A, et al. Preliminary findings: behavioral worsening on donepezil in patients with frontotemporal dementia. Am J Geriatr Psychiatry 2007;15(1):84–7.
43. McGleenon BM, Dynan KB, Passmore AP. Acetylcholinesterase inhibitors in Alzheimer's disease. Br J Clin Pharmacol 1999;48(4):471–80.
44. Kishi T, Matsunaga S, Oya K, et al. Memantine for alzheimer's disease: an updated systematic review and meta-analysis. J Alzheimers Dis 2017;60(2):401–25.
45. Reisberg B, Doody R, Stoffler A, et al. Memantine in moderate-to-severe Alzheimer's disease. N Engl J Med 2003;348(14):1333–41.
46. Orgogozo JM, Rigaud AS, Stoffler A, et al. Efficacy and safety of memantine in patients with mild to moderate vascular dementia: a randomized, placebo-controlled trial (MMM 300). Stroke 2002;33(7):1834–9.
47. McShane R, Westby MJ, Roberts E, et al. Memantine for dementia. Cochrane Database Syst Rev 2019;(3):CD003154.
48. Forbes D, Forbes SC, Blake CM, et al. Exercise programs for people with dementia. Cochrane Database Syst Rev 2015;(4):CD006489.
49. Panza GA, Taylor BA, MacDonald HV, et al. Can exercise improve cognitive symptoms of alzheimer's disease? J Am Geriatr Soc 2018;66(3):487–95.
50. Zou L, Loprinzi PD, Yeung AS, et al. The beneficial effects of mind-body exercises for people with mild cognitive impairment: a systematic review with meta-analysis. Arch Phys Med Rehabil 2019;100(8):1556–73.
51. Hill NT, Mowszowski L, Naismith SL, et al. Computerized cognitive training in older adults with mild cognitive impairment or dementia: a systematic review and meta-analysis. Am J Psychiatry 2017;174(4):329–40.
52. Woods B, Aguirre E, Spector AE, et al. Cognitive stimulation to improve cognitive functioning in people with dementia. Cochrane Database Syst Rev 2012;(2):CD005562.
53. Aguirre E, Woods RT, Spector A, et al. Cognitive stimulation for dementia: a systematic review of the evidence of effectiveness from randomised controlled trials. Ageing Res Rev 2013;12(1):253–62.
54. Wells RE, Kerr C, Dossett ML, et al. Can adults with mild cognitive impairment build cognitive reserve and learn mindfulness meditation? qualitative theme analyses from a small pilot study. J Alzheimers Dis 2019;70(3):825–42.
55. Penninkilampi R, Casey AN, Singh MF, et al. The association between social engagement, loneliness, and risk of dementia: a systematic review and meta-analysis. J Alzheimers Dis 2018;66(4):1619–33.

56. Sommerlad A, Sabia S, Singh-Manoux A, et al. Association of social contact with dementia and cognition: 28-year follow-up of the Whitehall II cohort study. PLoS Med 2019;16(8):e1002862.
57. Fancourt D, Steptoe A, Cadar D. Community engagement and dementia risk: time-to-event analyses from a national cohort study. J Epidemiol Community Health 2020;74(1):71–7.
58. Scarmeas N, Stern Y, Mayeux R, et al. Mediterranean diet and mild cognitive impairment. Arch Neurol 2009;66(2):216–25.
59. Cooper C, Sommerlad A, Lyketsos CG, et al. Modifiable predictors of dementia in mild cognitive impairment: a systematic review and meta-analysis. Am J Psychiatry 2015;172(4):323–34.
60. Droogsma E, van Asselt DZ, Scholzel-Dorenbos CJ, et al. Nutritional status of community-dwelling elderly with newly diagnosed Alzheimer's disease: prevalence of malnutrition and the relation of various factors to nutritional status. J Nutr Health Aging 2013;17(7):606–10.
61. Vancampfort D, Solmi M, Firth J, et al. The impact of pharmacologic and nonpharmacologic interventions to improve physical health outcomes in people with dementia: a meta-review of meta-analyses of randomized controlled trials. J Am Med Dir Assoc 2020. https://doi.org/10.1016/j.jamda.2020.01.010.
62. Kinnunen KM, Vikhanova A, Livingston G. The management of sleep disorders in dementia: an update. Curr Opin Psychiatry 2017;30(6):491–7.
63. Cassidy-Eagle E, Siebern A, Unti L, et al. Neuropsychological functioning in older adults with mild cognitive impairment and insomnia randomized to CBT-I or Control Group. Clin Gerontol 2018;41(2):136–44.
64. Perini G, Cotta Ramusino M, Sinforiani E, et al. Cognitive impairment in depression: recent advances and novel treatments. Neuropsychiatr Dis Treat 2019;15:1249–58.
65. Smith BC, D'Amico M. Sensory-based interventions for adults with dementia and alzheimer's disease: a scoping review. Occup Ther Health Care 2019;1–31. https://doi.org/10.1080/07380577.2019.1608488.
66. Kales HC, Gitlin LN, Lyketsos CG. Assessment and management of behavioral and psychological symptoms of dementia. BMJ 2015;350:h369.
67. Wilkins JM, Forester BP. Update on SSRI treatment for neuropsychiatric symptoms of dementia. Curr Psychiatry Rep 2016;18(2):14.
68. Sepehry AA, Lee PE, Hsiung GY, et al. Effect of selective serotonin reuptake inhibitors in Alzheimer's disease with comorbid depression: a meta-analysis of depression and cognitive outcomes. Drugs Aging 2012;29(10):793–806.
69. Koenig AM, Butters MA. Cognition in late life depression: treatment considerations. Curr Treat Options Psychiatry 2014;1(1):1–14.
70. Porsteinsson AP, Drye LT, Pollock BG, et al. Effect of citalopram on agitation in Alzheimer disease: the CitAD randomized clinical trial. JAMA 2014;311(7):682–91.
71. Funk KA, Bostwick JR. A comparison of the risk of QT prolongation among SSRIs. Ann Pharmacother 2013;47(10):1330–41.
72. Santa Cruz MR, Hidalgo PC, Lee MS, et al. Buspirone for the treatment of dementia with behavioral disturbance. Int Psychogeriatr 2017;29(5):859–62.
73. McDermott CL, Gruenewald DA. Pharmacologic management of agitation in patients with dementia. Curr Geriatr Rep 2019;8(1):1–11.
74. Kuehn BM. FDA warns antipsychotic drugs may be risky for elderly. JAMA 2005;293(20):2462.

75. Yohanna D, Cifu AS. Antipsychotics to treat agitation or psychosis in patients with dementia. JAMA 2017;318(11):1057–8.
76. Cummings J, Ballard C, Tariot P, et al. Pimavanserin: potential treatment for dementia-related psychosis. J Prev Alzheimers Dis 2018;5(4):253–8.
77. Cipriani G, Lucetti C, Danti S, et al. Sleep disturbances and dementia. Psycho-geriatrics 2015;15(1):65–74.
78. McCleery J, Cohen DA, Sharpley AL. Pharmacotherapies for sleep disturbances in dementia. Cochrane Database Syst Rev 2016;(11):CD009178.

Common Urinary and Bowel Disorders in the Geriatric Population

Zara Manuelyan, MD[a], Keila Siomara Muñiz, MD[b],
Ellen Stein, MD[a],*

KEYWORDS

- Gastrointestinal motility • Small intestinal bacterial overgrowth • Lactose intolerance
- Constipation • Irritable bowel syndrome • Diverticular disease • Fecal incontinence
- Lower urinary tract symptoms (LUTS)

KEY POINTS

- Urinary incontinence and lower urinary tract symptoms (LUTSs) can have a significant impact on a person's health as a result of the association with depression and anxiety, social isolation and embarrassment, sexual dysfunction, falls, and infections.
- Anticholinergic/antimuscarinic medications may be associated with a risk of cognitive impairment and caution should be taken when prescribing these to geriatric patients.
- LUTSs in older adults are treatable conditions and appropriate counseling and management can lead to significant improvements in quality of life.
- Constipation and fecal incontinence are common treatable conditions in elderly patients.

URINARY DISORDERS
Introduction

The prevalence of urinary incontinence and other lower urinary tract symptoms (LUTSs) increases with older age. Urinary symptoms are more noticeable in men after the seventh decade of life and in women after menopause. Changes in the lower urinary tract and the nervous system that support this observation are multifactorial and often incorrectly categorized as part of normal aging. LUTSs can have a significant impact on a person's health, including physical, psychological, and emotional or social well-being. This article summarizes the current literature regarding the occurrence of lower urinary tract symptoms in the geriatric population.

[a] Department of Gastroenterology, Johns Hopkins University School of Medicine, 4940 Eastern Avenue, 3rd Floor, A Building Johns Hopkins Bayview, Baltimore, MD 21224, USA;
[b] Department of Gynecology and Obstetrics, Johns Hopkins University School of Medicine, 4940 Eastern Avenue, 301 Building, Suite 3100, Baltimore, MD 21224, USA
* Corresponding author.
E-mail address: estein6@jhmi.edu

Med Clin N Am 104 (2020) 827–842
https://doi.org/10.1016/j.mcna.2020.06.009
0025-7125/20/© 2020 Elsevier Inc. All rights reserved.

Definitions

LUTSs can be grouped into 4 main categories[1]:

- Urinary incontinence symptoms.
- Bladder storage symptoms (including increased daytime urinary frequency, nocturia, urgency, and overactive bladder).
- Sensory symptoms or the departure from normal sensation or function experienced during bladder filling.
- Voiding and postmicturition symptoms, including changes in normal sensation or function during or following micturition, such as hesitancy, straining to void, incomplete bladder emptying.

The prevalence of many LUTSs, and in particular nocturia, urinary urgency, and urgency incontinence, increases with advancing age.

There are 3 main types of urinary incontinence. First, stress urinary incontinence (SUI), the involuntary loss of urine on effort, physical exertion, sneezing, or coughing. Second, urgency urinary incontinence (UUI) is the involuntary loss of urine associated with urgency, and often combines with the complaint of inability to reach the toilet in time. This symptom is typically caused by involuntary detrusor contractions. Mixed urinary incontinence describes signs and symptoms of both SUI and UUI. Frequency is the complaint of voiding too often. Urgency is the complaint of a sudden compelling desire to pass urine that is difficult to defer. Urgency can occur with or without incontinence. Nocturia is the complaint of waking at night 1 or more times to void. Third, overactive bladder syndrome (OAB) is urinary urgency, usually accompanied by frequency and nocturia, with or without incontinence, in the absence of a urinary tract infection or other obvious disorder. A less common subtype is overflow incontinence, which involves the involuntary loss of urine when the bladder does not empty completely, and is associated with high residual urine volumes or urinary retention.

Physiologic changes in the kidneys and bladder can predispose older adults with risk factors to developing LUTSs. Bladder sensation and contractility decrease with age. In men, the prostate enlarges, and, in women, sphincter strength and urethral length decrease.[2] Reduced urine production by the kidneys combined with increased bladder collagen content and involuntary bladder contractions can result in an increase in postvoid residual volume.[2] Thus, these physiologic changes combined with additional challenges that the geriatric population faces are important to keep in mind when caring for these patients.

DISCUSSION
Epidemiology

The most comprehensive longitudinal study of lower urinary tract symptoms in community-dwelling population 60 years of age and older is the Medical, Epidemiologic and Social Aspects of Aging (MESA) study.[3] MESA established the 24-hour urinary frequency and nocturnal urinary pattern in the elderly. Of 500 men 60 years of age and older studied, 36.2% without urinary symptoms of incontinence, bladder irritability, or difficulty emptying voided 4 to 5 times in a 24-hour period. Nearly 80% of these men had a frequency of 4 to 8 times throughout a 24-hour period. Only 12% voided more than 8 times per day and 8.2% voided 1 to 3 times per day. Among 560 asymptomatic women, 34.8% voided 4 to 5 times per day, 47.3% voided 6 to 8 times per day, 12.3% voided more than 8 times per day, and 5.5% voided fewer than 4 times per day. Among 400 asymptomatic men, 34.8% did not experience nocturia, 40.5% voided 1 time at night, 17.8% voided twice, and 6.9% voided 3 or more times at night.

Among 479 asymptomatic women, 37.2% did not experience nocturia, 38.8% voided 1 time at night, 16.7% voided 2 times, and 7.3% voided 3 or more times at night. The 24-hour urinary frequency and the nocturnal urinary pattern increased significantly in both men and women when there were associated urinary symptoms, such as incontinence, difficult bladder emptying, or bladder irritability. Specifically, in women with incontinence, approximately 30% voided 9 or more times in a 24-hour period and 41% voided 2 or more times at night.

Prevalence rates for urinary incontinence range from 8% to 34% in the geriatric population.[4] The prevalence of incontinence among women 60 years of age and older living in the community was 38% and, among men 60 years of age and older, it was 19%.[3] In a multinational cohort study,[5] prevalence of all LUTSs increased in association with increasing age, with 62.9% of men and 58.7% of women 60 years of age and older reporting any LUTSs. Similarly, an age-associated increase was observed in the prevalence of urinary urgency, from 7.1% in men and 9.7% in women less than 40 years of age to 19.1% in men and 18.3% in women 60 years of age and older. The prevalence of incontinence (of any cause) increased from 2.4% in men and 7.3% in women less than 40 years of age to 5.4% and 19.5%, respectively, in those 60 years of age and older. Similarly, the Norwegian Epidemiology of Incontinence in the County of Nord-Trøndelag (EPINCONT) study[6] described a cohort of 27,936 community-dwelling women with a 40% prevalence of urinary incontinence in those 90 years of age and older.

Furthermore, urinary incontinence prevalence among nearly 1000 85-year-old community-dwelling men and women in Goteborg, Sweden, was 29%,[7] whereas 84% of adults residing in nursing homes or hospitals experienced incontinence. Similar rates were found in Moscow and Malaysia.[8,9] In an American survey reporting on specific types of incontinence, the median age of women with urge incontinence was 61 years.[10] Stress incontinence was more common in younger women aged 30 to 49 years, 78% compared with 57% for those 50 to 89 years of age. Urge incontinence predominated in the older population, 67% compared with 56% in women less than 50 years of age.[11]

Impact on Health

Urinary incontinence and LUTSs can have a significant social impact, with associated depression, anxiety, social isolation, embarrassment, and sexual dysfunction.[12,13] Medical consequences of LUTSs in older adults include an increased risk of falls, occurring 1.5 to 2.3 times more often in older women with urinary urgency or urge incontinence,[14] as well as an increase in perineal and urinary tract infections (UTIs). UTIs are the second most common infection in geriatric populations.[15] Urinary incontinence, impaired cognitive function, and limited activity increase the susceptibility of the elderly to infections.[16] Furthermore, loss of independence and increased caregiver burden highlight the negative impact of LUTSs on the elderly.[17,18] From 6% to 10% of nursing home admissions in the United States are attributable to urinary incontinence.[19] The overall morbidity, mortality, and health care costs on older adults secondary to LUTSs have a profound impact on overall quality of life.

EVALUATION
History

Any evaluation for LUTSs should include a medical, surgical, and (for women) gynecologic history. Clinicians should elicit the patient's symptoms and severity, assess impact on quality of life, evaluate for comorbid conditions, and identify any reversible causes of urinary incontinence. A useful mnemonic for other causes of urinary incontinence is DIAPPERS (delirium, infection, atrophy, pharmacology, psychology, endocrinopathy, restricted mobility, and stool impaction). Women should also be evaluated for pelvic organ prolapse (POP).

Validated questionnaires can be used to elicit a symptom history, such as the International Consultation on Incontinence Questionnaire, Overactive Bladder Questionnaire, Pelvic Floor Distress Inventory, Urogenital Distress Inventory, Incontinence Severity Index, Incontinence Impact Questionnaire, Pelvic Floor Impact Questionnaire, and the POP/Urinary Incontinence Sexual Questionnaire. Bladder diaries are often useful tools in which the patient records the volume and frequency of fluid intake and voiding as well as symptoms of frequency and urgency and episodes of incontinence for at least 24 hours, and ideally for 2 to 3 days.

Diagnostic Tests

A urinalysis and/or urine culture can evaluate for microscopic hematuria or UTI as a cause of urinary symptoms. A postvoid residual (PVR) measurement can aid in diagnosing overflow incontinence or urinary retention. Most clinicians consider an abnormal PVR to be greater than 150 mL. If an increased PVR is identified, the test should be repeated.

Cystourethroscopy assesses the anatomy of bladder and urethra for abnormalities and the presence of foreign bodies. Urodynamic studies assess the physiologic function of the bladder during filling, storage, and voiding. Multichannel cystometrics can be used for patients with complex symptoms or voiding complaints. Urodynamic evaluation is not required in the assessment of all patients with urinary incontinence symptoms (even those planning for an anti-incontinence procedure) but should be considered as a tool to aid in diagnosis for certain patient populations. At-risk populations include prior history of incontinence surgery, history of pelvic radiation, failure to respond to treatments for incontinence, neurogenic voiding dysfunction, mixed incontinence symptoms, or concern for overflow incontinence.

TREATMENT
Conservative Treatment of Lower Urinary Tract Symptoms/Urinary Incontinence

Conservative treatment options for most types of LUTs, including OAB/UUI, SUI, or mixed incontinence, can be effective as initial strategies. Lifestyle modifications that are recommended include weight loss; avoidance of dietary irritants, including reduction of caffeine intake; smoking cessation; and management of daily fluid intake. Weight loss has been found to be more effective for stress incontinence than OAB/UUI but may be beneficial for both. Bladder retraining, which involves scheduled voiding with progressive increases in the interval between voids, and urge suppression techniques are effective for people with OAB/UUI. Prompted and scheduled voiding may be warranted in geriatric patients with cognitive impairment or difficulty with mobility. Pelvic floor muscle exercises (PFMEs) requiring repeated voluntary pelvic floor muscle training (ie, Kegel exercises), may be used in conjunction with bladder retraining. PFMEs performed in a supervised pelvic floor physical therapy program are more effective than exercises performed independently. In addition to PFMEs, fitness exercises have been found to be beneficial in improving incontinence in extremely frail and deconditioned nursing home residents.[20,21]

Nonsurgical Treatment of Stress Urinary Incontinence

Women can be fitted for a vaginal support device, known as a continence pessary, for SUI. Care of the pessary must be demonstrated. Pessaries can be used independently or in conjunction with PFME. Pharmacologic therapy is not recommended for SUI in men or women because of lack of efficacy and high rates of adverse side effects.

Surgical Treatment of Stress Urinary Incontinence

The midurethral sling is considered the gold standard procedure for treatment of SUI in women and can be placed via a minimally invasive retropubic or transobturator approach. Midurethral polypropylene mesh slings have been found to be as effective as other surgical procedures for SUI (eg, fascial slings or Burch colposuspension) with the benefit of shorter operative time and decreased morbidity,[22] which is especially significant when factoring in recovery time in older adults. Retropubic urethropexy procedures are now less commonly performed because of increased morbidity relative to the less invasive midurethral slings. These procedures include the Burch retropubic colposuspension and the Marshall-Marchetti-Krantz.

In men, the most common treatments for SUI are the artificial urinary sphincter (AUS) and a variety of male slings. The AUS was first introduced more than 30 years ago and is considered by many urologists to be the gold standard for male SUI treatment.[23]

Urethral bulking agent injections may be appropriate in patients with SUI with or without urethral hypermobility (ie, mobility of <30°) who are unwilling or unable to tolerate a surgical procedure.

Conservative Treatment of Overactive Bladder Syndrome

First-line treatment of OAB includes behavioral and lifestyle modifications, such as weight loss, avoidance of bladder irritants, PFMEs, and bladder retraining with or without pharmacotherapy. If these methods provide unsatisfactory results, advanced therapies can be pursued.

Medical Management of Overactive Bladder Syndrome

At present there are 2 classes of medications that are typically used for the treatment of OAB: anticholinergics/antimuscarinics and beta3-agonists. Medications may be combined with behavioral therapies to improve efficacy. Anticholinergics/antimuscarinics inhibit involuntary detrusor contractions and act primarily by increasing bladder capacity and decreasing urgency through blockade of muscarinic receptor stimulation by acetylcholine during bladder storage.[24] There are 6 antimuscarinic medications available in various formulations in the United States: darifenacin, fesoterodine, oxybutynin, solifenacin, tolterodine, and trospium. They have minimal differences in efficacy.

Dry mouth is the most common side effect, as well as dry eyes and constipation. These medications are not recommended in patients with closed-angle glaucoma or impaired gastric emptying. A large study showed an associated increased dementia risk in patients taking these anticholinergics/antimuscarinics.[25] Caution should be taken when prescribing anticholinergic medications in frail or cognitively impaired geriatric patients, and when needed using the lowest effective dose or alternatives.

Mirabegron is a beta3-agonist that relaxes the detrusor muscle during storage and increases bladder capacity by augmenting sympathetic nervous system stimulation of the bladder. Mirabegron should not be used in patients with uncontrolled hypertension but has an overall favorable side effect profile compared with anticholinergics. Antimuscarinic and beta3-agonist medications can be used together in patients with persistent symptoms who are unable to increase medication dose secondary to side effects or dose limits. In trials comparing mirabegron plus solifenacin in various dosage combinations with solifenacin alone, combination therapy resulted in improved OAB symptoms compared with either monotherapy dose.[26,27]

Tricyclic antidepressants such as imipramine improve bladder hypertonicity and compliance. Efficacy is not well established, and adverse effects are common, therefore imipramine is not commonly used for treatment of OAB.

Surgical Management of Overactive Bladder Syndrome

For patients who have failed conservative management or desire to avoid the side effects of medications, surgical management of OAB may be considered. Advanced therapies include sacral nerve root neuromodulation, posterior tibial nerve stimulation, and chemodenervation with intradetrusor injection of onabotulinumtoxinA. Invasive procedures such as augmentation cystoplasty or urinary diversion via an ileal conduit are reserved for severe refractory cases.

Treatment of Mixed Urinary Incontinence

Older adults with mixed urinary incontinence should be counseled that primary treatment of SUI does not treat UUI symptoms. Patients should be assessed to determine whether symptoms are stress or urge predominant, because this effects treatment. PFMEs, behavioral therapy, and lifestyle modifications can affect both types of incontinence, but treatment beyond these should be tailored to the patient's symptoms.

Clinics Care Points

- Physiologic changes in the kidneys and bladder can predispose older adults with risk factors to developing LUTSs.
- Urinary incontinence and LUTSs can have a significant impact on a person's health as a result of the association with depression and anxiety, social isolation and embarrassment, sexual dysfunction, falls, and infections.
- Conservative treatment options for most types of LUTs, including OAB/UUI, SUI, and mixed incontinence, can be effective as initial strategies. These strategies include weight loss and avoidance of dietary irritants, including reduction of caffeine intake, smoking cessation, and management of daily fluid intake.
- For patients with OAB and urgency incontinence, reliable evidence indicates that caution should be taken when prescribing anticholinergic medications in frail or cognitively impaired geriatric patients. Providers should prescribe the lowest effective dose or consider alternative medications in these high-risk elderly patients.
- Mirabegron, a beta3-agonist, should not be used in patients with uncontrolled hypertension, but has an overall favorable side effect profile compared with anticholinergics.

BOWEL DISORDERS
Introduction

Gastrointestinal (GI) and digestive disorders may occur at any age, but physiologic changes and decline related to aging lead to increased prevalence of these GI diseases in the elderly. Nearly 16% of the world population will be 65 years of age and older by the year 2050.[28] There are common GI bowel disorders affecting geriatric patients, and this article focuses on clinical characteristics, diagnostic tools, and management of bowel disorders.

Small Intestine

The functional capacity of the small intestine in the geriatric population is comparable with younger populations. In terms of small bowel motility, small bowel transit time in young adults is between 2 and 6 hours. There are few studies estimating the transit time in the elderly population, but patterns of motility seem to be unchanged during aging.[29] Animal models of mucosa show age-related differences in the small intestine, such as increase in villous height and crypt depth and decrease in the mucosal surface area, but no such changes were observed in the duodenum in the elderly population.[30,31] Hormone secretion and absorptive capabilities of the small bowel are also not significantly different in geriatric adults.[32] Physiologic changes with aging have shown altered absorption of calcium, zinc, and magnesium. Lactase-phlorizin hydrolase disaccharide enzyme is significantly reduced in function with advancing age. A study by Di Stefano and colleagues[33] showed subjects more than 74 years old with statistically significant lower lactose absorption using breath hydrogen analysis compared with younger subjects. Interestingly, elderly patients with malabsorption had fewer reported symptoms of lactose intolerance. In terms of mucosal immunity in the intestine, aging seems to be associated with reduced immunity. There is progressive decline in the production of antigen-specific immunoglobulin A in the elderly.[34,35] Bacterial and viral pathogens in the GI tract are more commonly seen in the elderly population and more frequently lead to complications compared with young adults.

Small intestinal bacterial overgrowth (SIBO) is defined as the presence of excess bacteria in the small bowel. The prevalence of SIBO is much higher in the geriatric compared with younger populations, 15.6% and 5.9%, respectively.[36] Factors that predispose the elderly to SIBO are achlorhydria, anatomic abnormalities such as bowel resection, and small intestinal dysmotility. Moreover, the risk of SIBO is increased in patients treated with proton pump inhibitors. Gastric emptying delay can also contribute to bacterial stasis in the GI tract. Other medical conditions that are associated with increased risk of SIBO are scleroderma, polymyositis, portal hypertension, chronic kidney disease, and diabetes. In a study by Haboubi and colleagues,[37] small intestinal biopsies from patients with SIBO showed blunting of intestinal villi, and increased levels of intraepithelial lymphocytes, which were reversed after antibiotic therapy. Classic symptoms of SIBO include nausea, vomiting, and diarrhea. The presenting symptoms in the elderly might be vague, with nonspecific symptoms of abdominal bloating and distension. Malabsorption, such as vitamin B_{12} deficiency, could be the first clue for SIBO in the geriatric population. Vitamin K and folic acid levels are normal in these patients because they are produced by the bacteria.[38,39] The simplest method to diagnose SIBO is breath testing using a carbohydrate such as lactulose or glucose. The exhaled gas (hydrogen and/or methane) produced by the bacterial metabolism is measured to perform the study.[40,41] Medical therapy consists of dietary modifications with a low-carbohydrate diet/low-FODMAP (fermentable, oligosaccharides, disaccharides, monosaccharides, and polyols) diet, prokinetic agents to improve GI motility, and antibiotic therapy to reduce the bacterial overload in the small bowel. In the elderly, antibiotic therapy needs to be used cautiously because of an increased risk of *Clostridium difficile* colitis and increased rates of complications of *C difficile* colitis. The benefits of adding new prokinetic medications should be weighed against the adverse effects of polypharmacy.

Large Intestine

Data on transit time in the colon in elderly patients are conflicting. Hanani and colleagues[42] examined myenteric ganglia in human colonic specimens between the ages of 10 days and 91 years and concluded that there are increased abnormalities in the human myenteric plexus with increasing age, which could be affecting the colonic motility in the elderly population. Southwell and colleagues[43] observed that, in the human sigmoid colon, there are reductions in the levels of neurotransmitters, such as nitric oxide and vasoactive intestinal peptide in the nerve fibers, with growth from the pediatric age group to late adolescence but no significant differences with aging in the healthy elderly group. Further studies will help reach a consensus regarding effects of aging on the function of the large intestine. It seems that comorbid conditions, lifestyle factors such as inactivity, polypharmacy, and medication side effects play a crucial role in development of constipation. The leading group of medications associated with constipation are opioids and anticholinergics.

Constipation can arise in all ages, and chronic constipation affects approximately 15% of the US general population.[44] Sonnenberg and Koch[45] observed the incidence of constipation in adults 65 years of age and older to be 30% to 40% as measured by symptom scales. The incidence increases when evaluating geriatric nursing home residents, with nearly 50% affected.[46] According to epidemiologic studies, increased prevalence of laxative use has been reported in the elderly, and up to 74% of elderly patients residing in long-term facilities are being treated with daily laxatives.[47] In the United States, constipation is more commonly seen in women with pelvic floor dysfunction as a consequence of childbirth and pelvic surgery.[48] Constipation is defined using the Rome IV criteria. To fulfill the criteria, patients must have at least 2 of the following symptoms during the last 3 months: fewer than 3 spontaneous bowel movements per week; straining, lumpy, or hard stools; sensation of anorectal blockage or obstruction; sensation of incomplete evacuation; manual maneuvering for facilitated defecation for more than 25% of defecation attempts.[49]

Primary constipation, also referred to as functional constipation, is subsequently divided into 3 subgroups: normal transit constipation, slow transit constipation, and anorectal dysfunction. Normal transit constipation is the most common type in the general population. In the elderly, slow transit constipation and anorectal dysfunction are more commonly seen. Slow transit constipation is defined as increased transit time of stool through the colon with decreased frequency of defecation caused by myopathy, abnormal innervations of the bowel, or evacuation disorders caused by dyssynergy. Anorectal dysfunction is caused by ineffective coordination of the pelvic musculature and poor evacuation technique leading to defecation difficulty. It has been observed that impaired rectal contractions, reductions in internal anal sphincter pressure, reduced pelvic muscle strength, and impaired rectal sensation in the elderly are the physiologic alterations responsible for worsening anorectal dysfunction.[50]

Secondary constipation is defined as a constipation caused by other medications or disorders. It may be a side effect of certain medications such as calcium channel blockers, opioids, or nonsteroidal antiinflammatory drugs, or associated with chronic disorders such as neurologic, endocrine, rheumatologic, or psychiatric conditions. Neurologic conditions include neurogenic bowel dysfunction caused by spinal cord injury, stroke, or multiple sclerosis; autoimmune disorders, such as scleroderma; and endocrine diseases, such as hypocalcemia and hypothyroidism. **Table 1** summarizes the commonly used medical agents for constipation and their potential adverse effects.

Irritable bowel syndrome (IBS) is a functional GI disorder estimated to affect about 10% to 20% of the elderly population.[51] IBS is diagnosed based on the Rome clinical criteria, currently now in version IV. IBS is defined as recurrent abdominal pain in the last 3 months that is associated with alterations in bowel movements, such as stool consistency, frequency, and appearance.[52] There are 4 different subtypes defined

Table 1
Medical management of constipation

Medical Options	Available Agents in Category	Cost	Adverse Potential Effects
Fiber	All psyllium supplements	$	Abdominal discomfort and bloating
Laxatives	Miralax	$	Diarrhea, dehydration
Stimulants and osmotics	Dulcolax Senna Lactulose Milk of Magnesia	$	Diarrhea, abdominal pain, nausea, vomiting, electrolyte disturbance Lactulose additional bloating, flatulence, dehydration
Secretagogues	Lubiprostone Linaclotide Plecanatide	$$$	Diarrhea, dehydration, electrolyte disturbance
Selective serotonin type 4 (5-HT4) receptor agonist	Prucalopride	$$$$	Headache, diarrhea, dizziness, nausea, bloating
Neurologic	Pyridostigmine	$	Twitching, muscle cramps, diarrhea, sweating, blurry vision
Novel phosphate	Tenapanor	$$$?	Diarrhea, abdominal distension, flatulence, dizziness
Enemas	Retrograde enemas Anterograde enemas Anal irrigation	$ $$ $$$	Irritation of anus and rectal area

Single dollar signs ($) indicate least expensive; multiple dollar signs indicate increasing expense.

based on bowel patterns, including constipation predominant (IBS-C), diarrhea predominant (IBS-D), IBS with mixed bowel habits, and unclassified.[53] Overall, few studies address IBS in elderly patients, and this means there is less information about these patients or about patients with coexisting cardiovascular, neurologic, and other comorbidities common to this group. IBS patterns are similar when comparing young and older patients. In older patients, systemic diseases, previous surgeries, medications, and their side effects can significantly alter the presentation.[54] For example, the prevalence of IBS-C subtype seems to be higher in the geriatric populations. The incidence of IBS is more frequent in adolescents, whereas it is infrequently diagnosed in the elderly. It is important for physicians to remember that older adults with new IBS symptoms may have another cause of the symptoms. Geriatric patients with new or worsening symptoms should have organic disorder excluded and undergo a comprehensive investigation to avoid missing a more serious diagnosis, such as bowel ischemia or malignancy. Management of IBS in the elderly includes lifestyle and dietary modifications such as a diet low in FODMAP and fiber supplementation. Cognitive behavior therapy has been shown to have great benefit in some patients. Pharmacologic intervention depends on the subtype of IBS. For IBS-C, patients are first treated with osmotic laxatives when fiber agents such as psyllium have failed, followed by secretagogues such as linaclotide or lubiprostone. Antidepressants such as tricyclics, selective serotonin reuptake inhibitors, and antispasmodics such as dicyclomine are used when trying to control pain as the predominant symptom.[55,56] In a meta-analysis, Black and colleagues[56] investigated 15 trials of secretagogues for

IBS-C and concluded that all drugs, including linaclotide, lubiprostone, plecanatide, and tenapanor, were superior to placebo and the efficacy was similar for all the drugs. Interestingly, IBS has been considered a functional disorder because of unclear pathogenesis, but there have been numerous studies in recent years showing inflammatory infiltration, more specifically mast cell hyperplasia and activation in the small and large bowel leading to visceral hypersensitivity and dysmotility. Park and colleagues[57] showed significant increase of mucosal mast cells in the terminal ileum, ascending colon, and rectum of patients with IBS-D compared with controls. In another study, Klooker and colleagues[58] performed a barostat study on 60 patients with IBS to analyze rectal sensitivity before and after 8 weeks of therapy randomized to either ketotifen or placebo. They were able to show that ketotifen significantly decreased abdominal pain and other symptoms of IBS, possibly pointing to stabilizing properties of the histamine receptor antagonist, ketotifen.[58]

Diverticular disease is prevalent in the elderly population, and the highest rates are seen in the Western world. With globalization, prevalence rates have increased in Asian populations as well. Current incidence is 50% of the population more than 70 years of age, and 66% in those more than 85 years of age.[59] Diverticular disease has a spectrum ranging from asymptomatic diverticula to complicated diverticulitis. There are 3 different stages of diverticular disease: asymptomatic; symptomatic uncomplicated, associated with chronic pain and diarrhea; and symptomatic complicated, associated with sepsis, bleeding, fistulization, and abscess formation.[60] Most patients with diverticulosis remain asymptomatic (80%–85%).[61] Clinical presentation of diverticular disease does not change with age, but its severity of episodes may vary from mild to moderate with inflammation, pain, and lower GI bleeding, and even to more severe features, including abscess formation and perforation. Traditional management incorporates bowel rest; antibiotic therapy; pain control; and, in select instances, surgical intervention. Acute diverticulitis responds to conservative therapy most of the time and patients are recommended to receive a colonoscopy 8 weeks after symptom resolution to exclude diverticular colitis or colon cancer. About 15% to 30% of cases need surgical intervention.[62] In terms of diverticular hemorrhage management, most elderly patients are treated nonoperatively with supportive care. Surgical intervention is needed if bleeding persists when medical, endoscopic, and angiographic techniques have failed. Blind resection in the elderly can be associated with higher rates of rebleeding (>60%) and mortality (>30%) from sepsis.[63]

Colorectal cancer (CRC) is the third leading cause of cancer and third cause of cancer death in the United States.[64] Overall, in the past decade there has been a significant decline in the CRC incidence and mortality because of increased CRC screening and surveillance.[65] The American Cancer Society estimates there will be 101,420 cases of colon cancer and 44,180 cases of rectal cancer diagnosed in the United States in 2019. The decreasing trend in colon cancer detection is noted in the populations of older adults, who previously had the highest observed risk of CRC. The increasing incidence of colon cancer in younger adults (<55 years old) has prompted new guidelines to suggest CRC screening begin at 45 years of age.[64,65]

CRC presentations can vary. The most common symptoms in the elderly between the ages of 65 and 79 years are change in caliber of stool, GI bleeding, constipation, and abdominal pain. Weight loss is also seen, but is more common in the age group more than 80 years of age. Adenomatous and advanced polyps with villous and tubulovillous features, size larger than 10 mm, with high-grade dysplasia have an increased prevalence in the older age group.[66] Moreover, right-sided polyps along with other types of polyps, such as sessile serrated adenomas, have been linked with increasing age.[67] The guidelines related to screening patients older than 85 years has become a complex, multifactorial discussion. At present, the US Preventive Service Task Force recommends cessation of screening in patients greater than 85 years old for CRC. They also recommend against screening for CRC between the ages of 76 and 85 years, with some modifications based on the individual patient.[68] Ongoing CRC screening in older patients should take into account risks and benefits of further screening based on the individual patient's goals of care, comorbidities, life expectancy, and functional status.[69,70] When life expectancy is less than 10 years, CRC screening should not be performed and the reasoning documented in the record. After the shared decision making about whether to screen, CRC screening types may be reviewed and a plan for follow-up of a positive finding should be discussed. More invasive testing options include colonoscopy, sigmoidoscopy, capsule colonoscopy, and computed tomographic colonography. Noninvasive options include stool-based tests: guaiac fecal occult blood test (FOBT), fecal immunochemical test (FIT), stool DNA testing, and blood testing. In the elderly, noninvasive testing has increased false-positive rates and therefore it is crucial to discuss the possibility of a need for invasive testing with a colonoscopy in these scenarios. In the right patients, FOBT and FIT provide an easier alternative in the elderly between the ages of 75 and 85 years or older and, if the results are negative, provides a less risky method of testing compared with the invasive options.[71,72] It is worth mentioning that recent studies have shown that CRC resection in geriatric patients is not associated with higher incidence of postsurgical mortality or complications, or reduced survival rates.[73–75]

Fecal incontinence (FI) is another common problem among the older age group. It is a health issue that leads to significant distress with serious impact and interference with daily activities and quality of life. The overall prevalence of FI increases with age from 2.6% to 15.3% when comparing patient populations between the ages of 20 to 29 years and greater than 70 years, respectively. The nursing home population encompasses 40% to 50% of residents with FI. Because of obstetric history, FI seems to affect more women than men in the younger populations, but, with age, the difference in prevalence becomes tapered with women (8.9%) and men (7.7%).[76,77] Factors and physiologic changes that lead to bowel incontinence include anal sphincter muscle weakness and sensory abnormalities, history of anorectal surgeries, rectal prolapse, rectocele, chronic constipation, and fecal impaction, as well as immobility and dementia.[78] In order to diagnose this condition, detailed history and physical examination should be conducted by the physician. Many primary care physicians do not ask the difficult questions or document symptoms related to FI in the medical record, which leads to a higher number of undiagnosed and untreated patients.[79,80] Further testing might include stool studies to identify an infectious cause, colonoscopy or anoscopy to evaluate the mucosa, anorectal manometry, and MRI defecography. As noted by Leung and colleagues,[80] impaired sphincter function, decreased rectal sensation, and sphincter dyssynergia, a risk factor for constipation and fecal impaction, were observed in high magnitudes in nursing home residents with the complaint of incontinence. Treatment options include dietary modifications, bulking agents to enhance stool consistency, and pelvic floor muscle training with physical therapy with or without biofeedback. A placebo-controlled randomized clinical trial by Bliss and colleagues[81] showed psyllium fiber supplementation increasing stool bulking compared with other types of fiber via fermentation in the colon, therefore improving FI. Moreover, a randomized clinical trial evaluating loperamide versus psyllium fiber for management of FI resulted in no significant difference between the groups, but noted improvement of FI episodes and severity in each group. Loperamide was associated with more side effects, such as constipation, with 29% versus 10% in the psyllium group.[82] In another randomized trial, Jelovsek and colleagues[83] studied 300 women randomly assigned to different treatments (loperamide, exercises, biofeedback). The study suggested that there are no significant differences between loperamide compared with placebo, anal exercises with biofeedback compared with educational pamphlet, loperamide combined with biofeedback versus placebo and biofeedback, or loperamide combined with an educational pamphlet. The combination of the first-line medical therapies as well as exercise and biofeedback interventions can help guide the therapy for FI. The role of biofeedback and anal exercises is under-recognized for the effective management of FI symptoms.[83]

Summary

Urinary conditions are likely to increase in prevalence because of the growth of the older population. Patients may be reluctant to initiate discussions about their incontinence and urinary symptoms because of embarrassment, lack of knowledge about treatment options, or fear of surgery. Thus, responsibility for initiating conversations about urinary problems must rest with medical professionals to ensure that as many older adults as possible receive appropriate care.

Bowel conditions increase in prevalence in the elderly because of intrinsic changes in the physiology of the gut with normal aging. FI is a particularly challenging disorder, leading to social isolation and reduction in quality of life. Like urinary dysfunction, bowel disorders cause symptoms and contribute to poor quality of life in the elderly. There is a need for greater attention to bowel dysfunction in the elderly, and the benefits of exercise and physiotherapy to restore or maintain function in elderly patients are particularly underused. Given the increasing elderly population, management of these disorders will be important for their future.

CLINICS CARE POINTS

- Older patients have significantly lower lactose absorption compared with younger patients.
- Diverticular disease is prevalent in the elderly population, and highest in Western populations.
- Ongoing CRC screening in older patients should take into account risks and benefits of further screening based on the individual patient's goals of care, comorbidities, life expectancy, and functional status
- FI is a common problem among the older age group, asking questions is critical to finding cases.

DISCLOSURE

The authors have nothing to disclose.

REFERENCES

1. Haylen BT, de Ridder D, Freeman RM, et al. An International Urogynecological Association (IUGA)/International Continence Society (ICS) joint report on the terminology for female pelvic floor dysfunction. Int Urogynecol J 2010;21:5–26.

2. Gibson W, Wagg A. Incontinence in the elderly, 'normal' ageing, or unaddressed pathology? Nat Rev Urol 2017;14(7):440–8.

3. Diokno AC, Brock BM, Brown MB, et al. Prevalence of urinary incontinence and other urological symptoms in the noninstitutionalized elderly. J Urol 1986;136:1022.

4. Herzog AR, Fultz NH. Prevalence and incidence of urinary incontinence in community-dwelling populations. J Am Geriatr Soc 1990;38:273.

5. Irwin DE, Milsom I, Hunskaar S, et al. Population-based survey of urinary incontinence, overactive bladder, and other lower urinary tract symptoms in five countries: results of the EPIC study. Eur Urol 2006;50(6):1306–14 [discussion: 1314–5].

6. Hannestad YS, Rortveit G, Sandvik H, et al. A community-based epidemiological survey of female urinary incontinence: the Norwegian EPINCONT study. J Clin Epidemiol 2000;53(11):1150–7.

7. Hellstrom L, Ekelund P, Milsom I, et al. The prevalence of urinary incontinence and use of incontinence aids in 85-year-old men and women. Age Ageing 1990;19:383.

8. Tkacheva ON, Runikhina NK, Ostapenko VS, et al. Prevalence of geriatric syndromes among people aged 65 years and older at four community clinics in Moscow. Clin Interv Aging 2018;13:251–9.

9. Murukesu RR, Singh DKA, Shahar S. Urinary incontinence among urban and rural community dwelling older women: prevalence, risk factors and quality of life. BMC Public Health 2019;19(Suppl 4):529.

10. Kinchen K, Bump RC, Gobier JR. Prevalence and frequency of stress urinary incontinence among community-dwelling women. Eur Urol 2002;(Suppl 1):85.

11. Luber KM, Boero S, Choe JY, et al. The demographics of pelvic floor disorders: currents observation and future projections. Am J Obstet Gynecol 2001;184:1496–501 [discussion: 1501–3].

12. Coyne KS, Sexton CC, Irwin DE, et al. The impact of overactive bladder, incontinence and other lower urinary tract symptoms on quality of life, work productivity, sexuality and emotional well-being in men and women: results from the EPIC study. BJU Int 2008;101:1388.

13. Coyne KS, Wein AJ, Tubaro A, et al. The burden of lower urinary tract symptoms: evaluating the effect of LUTS on health-related quality of life, anxiety and depression: EpiLUTS. BJU Int 2009;103(Suppl 3):4.

14. Gibson W, Hunter KF, Camicioli R, et al. The association between lower urinary tract symptoms and falls: Forming a theoretical model for a research agenda. Neurourol Urodyn 2018;37:501.

15. Pawelec G. Immunity and ageing in man. Exp Gerontol 2006;41(12):1239–42.

16. Tal S, Guller V, Levi S, et al. Profile and prognosis of febrile elderly patients with bacteremic urinary tract infection. J Infect 2005;50(4):296–305.

17. Schumpf LF, Theill N, Scheiner DA, et al. Urinary incontinence and its association with functional physical and cognitive health among female nursing home residents in Switzerland. BMC Geriatr 2017;17:17.

18. Gotoh M, Matsukawa Y, Yoshikawa Y, et al. Impact of urinary incontinence on the psychological burden of family caregivers. Neurourol Urodyn 2009;28:492.

19. Morrison A, Levy R. Fraction of nursing home admissions attributable to urinary incontinence. Value Health 2006;9:272.

20. Schnelle JF, MacRae PG, Ouslander JG, et al. Functional incidental training, mobility performance, and incontinence care with nursing home residents. J Am Geriatr Soc 1995;43:1356–62.

21. Kim H, Yoshida H, Suzuki T. The effects of multidimensional exercise treatment on community-dwelling elderly Japanese women with stress, urge, and mixed urinary incontinence: a randomized controlled trial. Int J Nurs Stud 2001;48:1165–72.

22. Ford AA, Rogerson L, Cody JD, et al. Mid-urethral sling operations for stress urinary in-continence in women. Cochrane Database Syst Rev 2015;(7):CD006375.

23. Lai HH, Hsu EI, Teh BS, et al. 13 years of experience with artificial urinary sphincter implantation at Baylor College of Medicine. J Urol 2007;177:1021–5.

24. Finney SM, Andersson KE, Gillespie JI, et al. Antimuscarinic drugs in detrusor overactivity and the overactive bladder syndrome: motor or sensory actions? BJU Int 2006;98:503.

25. Coupland CAC, Hill T, Dening T, et al. Anticholinergic drug exposure and the risk of dementia: a nested case-control study. JAMA Intern Med 2019;179(8):1084–93.

26. Drake MJ, Chapple C, Esen AA, et al. Efficacy and safety of mirabegron add-on therapy to solifenacin in incontinent overactive bladder patients with an inadequate response to initial 4-week solifenacin monotherapy: a randomised double-blind multicentre phase 3B study (BESIDE). Eur Urol 2016;70:136.

27. Abrams P, Kelleher C, Staskin D, et al. Combination treatment with mirabegron and solifenacin in patients with overactive bladder: exploratory responder analyses of efficacy and evaluation of patient-reported outcomes from a randomized, double-blind, factorial, dose-ranging, Phase II study (SYMPHONY). World J Urol 2017;35:827.

28. Global Issues Overview; Ageing In: United Nations. 2019. Available at: https://www.un.org/en/sections/issues-depth/ageing/. Accessed January 25th, 2020.

29. Madsen JL, Graff J. Effects of ageing on gastrointestinal motor function. Age Ageing 2004;33:154–9.

30. Ren WY, Wu KF, Li X, et al. Age-related changes in small intestinal mucosa epithelium architecture and epithelial tight junction in rat models. Aging Clin Exp Res 2014;26:183–91.

31. Lipski PS, Bennett MK, Kelly PJ, et al. Ageing and duodenal morphometry. J Clin Pathol 1992;45:450–2.

32. D'Souza AL. Ageing and the gut. Postgrad Med J 2007;83(975):44–53.

33. Di Stefano M, Veneto G, Malservis S. Lactose malabsorption and intolerance in the elderly. Scand J Gastroenterol 2001;36(12):1274–8.

34. Mabbott NA, Kobayashi A, Sehgal A, et al. Aging and the mucosal immune system in the intestine. Biogerontology 2015;16:133–45.

35. Santiago AF, Alves AC, Oliveira RP, et al. Aging correlates with reduction in regulatory-type cytokines and T cells in the gut mucosa. Immunobiology 2011;216:1085–93.

36. Parlesak A, Klein B, Schecher K, et al. Prevalence of small bowel bacterial overgrowth and its association with nutrition intake in nonhospitalized older adults. J Am Geriatr Soc 2003;51:768–73.

37. Haboubi NY, Lee GS, Montgomery RD. Duodenal mucosal morphometry of elderly patients with small intestinal bacterial overgrowth: Response to antibiotics treatment. Age Ageing 1991;20:29–32.

38. Suter PM, Golner BB, Goldin BR, et al. Reversal of protein-bound vitamin B12 malabsorption with antibiotics in atrophic gastritis. Gastroenterology 1991;101:1039–45.

39. Camilo E, Zimmerman J, Mason JB, et al. Folate synthesized by bacteria in the human upper small intestine is assimilated by the host. Gastroenterology 1996;110:991–8.

40. Walters B, Vanner SJ. Detection of bacterial overgrowth in IBS using the lactulose breath test: comparison with 14C-D-xylose and healthy controls. Am J Gastroenterol 2005;100(7):1566–70.

41. King CE, Toskes PP. Comparison of the 1 gram 14C-D-xylose, 10 gram lactulose and 80 gram glucose H2 breath test in patients with small intestinal bacterial overgrowth. Gastroenterology 1986;91:1447–51.

42. Hanani M, Fellig Y, Udassin R, et al. Age related changes in the morphology of the myenteric plexus of the human colon. Auton Neurosci 2004;113(1-2):71–8.
43. Southwell BR, Koh TL, Wong SQ, et al. Decrease in nerve fibre density in human sigmoid colon circular muscle occurs with growth but not aging. Neurogastroenterol Motil 2010;22:439–45.e6.
44. Staats PS, Markowitz J, Schein J. Incidence of constipation associated with long-acting opioid therapy: a comparative study. South Med J 2004;97(2):129–34.
45. Sonnenberg A, Koch TR. Epidemiology of constipation in the United States. Dis Colon Rectum 1989 Jan;32(1):1–8.
46. Phillips C, Polakoff D, Maue SK, et al. Assessment of constipation management in long-term care patients. J Am Med Dir Assoc 2001;2(4):149–54.
47. Vazquez RM, Bouras EP. Epidemiology and management of chronic constipation in elderly patients. Clin Interv Aging 2015;10:919–30.
48. Bannister JJ, Abouzekry L, Read NW. Effect of aging on anorectal function. Gut 1987;28:353–7.
49. Simren M, Palsson OS, Whitehead WE. Update on Rome IV criteria for colorectal disorders: implications for clinical practice. Curr Gastroenterol Rep 2017;19(4):15.
50. Bouras EP, Tangalos EG. Chronic constipation in the elderly. Gastroenterol Clin North Am 2009;38(3):463–80.
51. Canavan C, West J, Card T. The epidemiology of irritable bowel syndrome. Clin Epidemiol 2014;6:71–80.
52. Lacy BE, Patel NK. Rome criteria and a diagnostic approach to irritable bowel syndrome. J Clin Med 2017;6(11):99.
53. Bhattarai Y, Muniz Pedrogo DA, Kashyap PC. Irritable bowel syndrome: a gut microbiota-related disorder? Am J Physiol Gastrointest Liver Physiol 2017;312(1):G52–62.
54. Ahn J, Ehrenpreis ED. Emerging treatments for irritable bowel syndrome. Expert Opin Pharmacother 2002;3(1):9–21.
55. Moayyedi P, Mearin F, Azpiroz F, et al. Irritable bowel syndrome diagnosis and management: A simplified algorithm for clinical practice. United European Gastroenterol J 2017;5(6):773–88.
56. Black CJ, Burr NE, Quigley EM, et al. Efficacy of secretagogues in patients with irritable bowel syndrome with constipation: systematic review and network meta-analysis. Gastroenterology 2018;155(6):1753–63.
57. Park JH, Rhee P-L, Kim HS, et al. Mucosal mast cell counts correlate with visceral hypersensitivity in patients with diarrhea predominant irritable bowel syndrome. J Gastroenterol Hepatol 2006;21(1):71–8.
58. Klooker TK, Braak B, Koopman KE, et al. The mast cell stabiliser ketotifen decreases visceral hypersensitivity and improves intestinal symptoms in patients with irritable bowel syndrome. Gut 2010;59(9):1213–21.
59. Farrell RJ, Farrell JJ, Morrin MM. Diverticular disease in the elderly. Gastroenterol Clin North Am 2001;30(2):475–96.
60. Sheth AA, Longo W, Floch MH. Diverticular disease and diverticulitis. Am J Gastroenterol 2008;103(6):1550–6.
61. Stollman N, Raskin JB. Diverticular disease of the colon. Lancet 2004;363(9409):631–9.
62. Ferzoco LB, Raptopoulos V, Silen W. Acute diverticulitis. N Engl J Med 1998;338:1521–6.
63. Colombo PL, Todde A, Belisomo M, et al. Massive hemorrhage caused by colonic diverticulosis. Ann Ital Chir 1994;65:89–97.

64. Cancer Facts & Figures 2019. American Cancer Society. Available at: https://www.cancer.org/content/dam/cancer-org/research/cancer-facts-and-statistics/annual-cancer-facts-and-figures/2019/cancer-facts-and-figures-2019.pdf. Accessed July 7, 2020.

65. Siegel RL, Fedewa SA, Anderson WF, et al. Colorectal Cancer Incidence Patterns in the United States, 1974–2013. JNCI. J Natl Cancer Inst 2017;109(8).

66. Lieberman DA, Williams JL, Holub JL, et al. Race, ethnicity, and sex affect risk for polyps >9 mm in average-risk individuals. Gastroenterology 2014;147(2):351–8 [quiz: e314–55].

67. Omata F, Brown WR, Tokuda Y, et al. Modifiable risk factors for colorectal neoplasms and hyperplastic polyps. Intern Med 2009;48(3):123–8.

68. Available at: https://www.uspreventiveservicestaskforce.org/Page/Document/UpdateSummaryFinal/colorectal-cancer-screening. Accessed July 7, 2020.

69. McClymont KM, Lee SJ, Schonberg MA, et al. Usefulness and effect of online prognostic calculators. J Am Geriatr Soc 2014;62(12):2444–5.

70. Ko CW, Sonnenberg A. Comparing risks and benefits of colorectal cancer screening in elderly patients. Gastroenterology 2005;129(4):1163–70.

71. Levin B, Lieberman DA, McFarland B, et al. American Cancer Society Colorectal Cancer Advisory Group; US Multi-Society Task Force; American College of Radiology Colon Cancer Committee. Screening and surveillance for the early detection of colorectal cancer and adenomatous polyps, 2008: a joint guideline from the American Cancer Society, the US Multi-Society Task Force on Colorectal Cancer, and the American College of Radiology. Gastroenterology 2008;134(5):1570–95.

72. Nee J, Chippendale RZ, Feuerstein JD. Screening for colon cancer in older adults: risks, benefits, and when to stop. Mayo Clin Proc 2020;95(1):184–96.

73. Basso SM, Lumachi F, Pianon P, et al. Analysis of factors affecting short-term results in elderly patients undergoing elective surgical resection for stage I-II colon cancer. Anticancer Res 2017;37:1971–4.

74. Yen C, Simillis C, Choudhry M, et al. A comparative study of short-term outcomes of colorectal cancer surgery in the elderly population. Acta Chir Belg 2017;117(5):303–7.

75. British Colorectal Collaborative Group. Surgery for colorectal cancer in elderly patients: a systematic review. Lancet 2000;356:968–74.

76. Whitehead WE, Borrud L, Goode PS, et al. Fecal incontinence in US adults: epidemiology and risk factors. Gastroenterology 2009;137:512–7.

77. Leung FW, Schnelle JF. Urinary and fecal incontinence in nursing home residents. Gastroenterol Clin North Am 2008;37(3):697.

78. Tariq SH, Morley JE, Prather CM. Fecal incontinence in the elderly patient. Am J Med 2003;115(3):217–22.

79. Dunivan GC, Heymen S, Palsson OS, et al. Fecal incontinence in primary care: prevalence, diagnosis, and health care utilization. Am J Obstet Gynecol 2010;202:493.e1-e6.

80. Leung FW, Schnelle JF. Urinary and fecal incontinence in nursing home residents. Gastroenterol Clin North Am 2008;37(3):697.

81. Bliss DZ, Savik K, Jung HJ, et al. Dietary fiber supplementation for fecal incontinence: a randomized clinical trial. Res Nurs Health 2014;37:367–78.

82. Markland AD, Burgio KL, Whitehead WE, et al. Loperamide versus psyllium fiber for treatment of fecal incontinence. Dis Colon Rectum 2015;58(10):983–93.

83. Jelovsek JE, Markland AD, Whitehead WE, et al. Controlling faecal incontinence in women by performing anal exercises with biofeedback or loperamide: a randomised clinical trial. Lancet Gastroenterol Hepatol 2019;4(9):698–710.

Sadness and Worry in Older Adults

Differentiating Psychiatric Illness from Normative Distress

Julie Lutz, PhD, Kimberly A. Van Orden, PhD*

KEYWORDS

- Depression • Anxiety • Suicide • Grief • Bereavement • Social connectedness
- Social isolation • Geriatrics

KEY POINTS

- Later life is generally associated with greater emotional well-being.
- However, in certain contexts older adults may be more at risk for bereavement and grief, social isolation and loneliness, and suicide.
- Self-reported symptoms of depression and anxiety may differ for older adults, necessitating developmentally appropriate assessment of symptoms.
- It is critical to consider the balance of risk and resilience factors for depression and anxiety in late life, as well as developmental trajectories, rather than assessing each factor in isolation.

INTRODUCTION, BACKGROUND, AND DEFINITIONS

Although later life is broadly associated with greater emotional well-being,[1] older adults face a number of developmental changes that have the potential to negatively impact their mood and emotional well-being. This dichotomy between emotional well-being and emotional vulnerability in late life may be demonstrated by the relatively low rates of depression in this age group[2] compared with the fact that older men compose the demographic group with the highest risk of suicide in the United States[3] and around the world.[4] Further, older adults may present with a different array of risk factors and symptoms of depression or anxiety than younger adults.[2,5] Additionally, older adults may be at greater risk for changes that may frequently be comorbid with, but do not automatically confer a diagnosis of, depression or anxiety, such as grief, social isolation and/or loneliness, and thoughts of death. The aim of this review is to distinguish these phenomena from each other and from a major depressive disorder or

Department of Psychiatry, University of Rochester Medical Center, Center for the Study and Prevention of Suicide, 300 Crittenden Boulevard, Box PSYCH, Rochester, NY 14642, USA
* Corresponding author.
E-mail address: Kimberly_Vanorden@URMC.Rochester.edu
Twitter: @kimvanorden (K.A.V.O.)

Med Clin N Am 104 (2020) 843–854
https://doi.org/10.1016/j.mcna.2020.05.001

anxiety disorder in late life, to clarify normative and non-normative changes in emotional well-being among older adults, and to provide recommendations for assessment and intervention.

There is a common misconception of aging that depression or poor emotional well-being is common, or even normal, in late life.[6,7] This notion likely stems from a societal ageist bias, and beliefs that it is normal for late life to be characterized by poor health and poor functioning and, therefore, poor mental health.[7,8] It additionally stems from a lack of understanding of normative developmental changes throughout adulthood and late life. Emotional experiences can be understood in a developmental context, such that certain experiences are normative at certain times in life, whereas others are not normative in certain contexts. Without an understanding of these contexts, a developmentally normal experience may be mistaken to be pathologic, whereas an experience of suffering may be overlooked owing to an incorrect assumption that it is typical of a certain age. With greater knowledge of the developmental trajectory of emotional well-being in late life, a clinician may more accurately assess whether a patient's experience represents a divergence from a healthy trajectory, and what interventions may support that patient in getting back "on track."

For the purpose of this review, "normative" refers to phenomena appearing in research to be developmentally appropriate, or to occur among a large portion of the population without diagnosable mental illness. "Non-normative" refers to phenomena that are associated with maladaptive coping or adjustment, and possibly (but not necessarily) mental illness, that may be the target of intervention/treatment. The terms "depression" and "anxiety" refer to diagnosable disorders per the *Diagnostic and Statistical Manual of Mental Disorders* (DSM) 5th edition[9] and/or *International Classification of Diseases*, 10th edition,[10] such as major depressive disorder, generalized anxiety disorder, and so on. There will also be some discussion of subthreshold syndromes, in which an older adult may not meet criteria for a disorder, but experiences some symptoms with a significant effect on his or her quality of life.

NORMATIVE EMOTIONAL DEVELOPMENT IN LATE LIFE

Research to date on lifespan development has shown that, generally, later life is associated with greater emotional well-being, including less frequent negative affect and more frequent positive affect, and decreased lability in emotions.[1,11] One prominent theory posited to explain this phenomenon is the socioemotional selectivity theory.[12] The socioemotional selectivity theory posits that, as the end of life is perceived to draw nearer, people shift their goals from the acquisition of knowledge or exploration of new experiences, to the regulation of emotion and enhancement of positive emotional and relational experiences. In other words, as people perceive their time becoming more limited, they focus more on maximizing positive emotional states and minimizing negative emotional states in the present, often via seeking out stable and positive social contexts.

Taking a more expanded view by considering the age-related physiologic factors in emotional experience in addition to the psychological factors, the strength and vulnerability integration theory posits that later life is associated with both psychological enhancements in adaptive emotion regulation strategies (as described in the socioemotional selectivity theory) as well as physiologic vulnerabilities to situations involving higher, more prolonged negative emotional arousal.[13] With age, people build and hone effective psychological strategies for regulating average, common emotional experiences, therefore leading to a decrease in exposure to negative emotional experiences, improved ability to rebound after minor negative experiences, and a general increase in emotional well-being. However, aging is also associated with decreased physiologic flexibility and resilience, leaving older adults more vulnerable to distress when they experience high levels of physical arousal associated with an un-avoidable, prolonged state of stress or negative emotional arousal.

In behavioral and imaging studies of the brain as people age, patterns of resilience to negative emotional experience and reactivity to positive emotional experience are borne out, despite the general reality of physiologic and cognitive decline in later life.[14] Older adults exhibit less reactivity to negative stimuli, and greater memory for positive information. However, older adults who have damage to areas of the prefron-tal cortex related to emotion regulation are more likely to experience negative out-comes such as depression.[14]

These results indicate that, contrary to a common misconception that growing older is associated with a decline in emotional well-being,[6] the majority of older adults will experience a general improvement in emotional well-being in late life. However, older adults who are exposed to significant, unavoidable, prolonged stressors may be espe-cially vulnerable to negative outcomes, such as mood or anxiety disorders, or even suicidal thoughts or behaviors.

MOOD AND ANXIETY DISORDERS IN LATE LIFE

Numerous studies have documented that older adults have a lower prevalence of mood and anxiety disorders than younger adults,[15–17] which may be accounted for, in part, by increased levels of emotional well-being in later life. However, many believe that these estimates can be misleading, owing to issues of accurately detecting depression and anxiety in this population.[18] Under-recognition may occur due to underreporting of symptoms by older adults owing to stigma, or internalized ageism whereby older adults—and providers—expect depressed mood to accompany aging and thus do not think it warrants treatment. Physicians and other clinicians are less likely to ask older adults about psychological symptoms, including suicide ideation, than for younger adults.[18,19]

Older adults' presentation of mood or anxiety disorders often differ from younger adults, meaning that the symptoms older adults experience and describe differ from those of younger patients. Older adults are less likely to report sad or depressed mood, but more likely to report anhedonia (lack of pleasure),[5] apathy, and irritability.[20] In addition, older adults are more likely to describe somatic symptoms as their primary concern, such as those related to sleep, fatigue, and psychomotor slowing, as well as cognitive symptoms such as deficits in memory, concentration, processing speed, and executive functioning.[2] Depression in late life commonly co-occurs with gastroin-testinal and other somatic symptoms.[20] Older adults may also be more likely to pre-sent with a subthreshold depression, meaning that clinically significant depression symptoms are present, but not enough symptoms to meet the criteria for a major depressive episode. The clinical importance of subthreshold syndromes should not be minimized, because this syndrome is associated with a greater odds of lifetime psychiatric disorders and of developing major depressive disorder or an anxiety dis-order in the subsequent years.[21] Finally, because older adults are more likely to expe-rience multiple health problems, differentiating a depressive disorder from an underlying medical condition is essential and can be complex. Nonspecific physical symptoms, such as fatigue, loss of appetite, weakness, diffuse physical pain, and sleep problems, can be signs of a depressive illness or symptoms of an underlying medical condition. Depressive disorders and medical illnesses also frequently co-occur (and share symptoms) and can increase risk in both directions—a depressive disorder is associated with poor health and many medical illnesses are associated with increased risk for a depressive disorder.[2]

Older adults' presentations of anxiety disorders may differ somewhat from those of younger adults, including the topics of worry (eg, more concerns about health and fewer about work or school),[5,22] but there are fewer differences than regarding depression. Older and younger adults report comparable symptoms of anxiety disorders, but they may describe their symptoms differently, using terms such as "stressed" or "tense" rather than "anxious," "worried," or "nervous."[5] Given these differences in the presentation of anxiety in late life, recommendations for future diagnostic classifications have included attention to the heterogeneity of anxiety symptoms and experiences in older adults, the use of language appropriate to the older adult in the assessment of anxiety, consideration of comorbidities (eg, comorbid depression, medical illness, and cognitive impairment), and attention to variants of anxiety that are mostly exclusive to late life (eg, fear of falling).[23]

As clinicians assess for the presence of mood or anxiety disorders among older adults, they should be alert to these possible differences in presentation and use appropriate assessment strategies and instruments. The use of assessment instruments developed and validated specifically for use in older adults (eg, Geriatric Depression Scale,[24] Geriatric Anxiety Inventory[25]) is recommended, because such instruments take into account differences in symptom presentations and measurement in older adults and are designed to be easy to administer, with yes/no response choices. Additionally, best judgment should be used regarding the presence of distressing subthreshold mood symptoms that may merit an intervention, although they may not meet diagnostic criteria.

BEREAVEMENT AND GRIEF

Losses become a normative part of life in older adulthood, including bereavement (death of a loved one) and loss of prior levels of health and physical functioning. However, although loss is a common experience in later life, that does not mean that all grief reactions will resolve on their own or do not warrant intervention. For example, individuals who have experienced bereavement are at greater risk for declines in health and functioning, potentially increased risk of mortality, decline in socioemotional well-being, and increase in loneliness and social isolation.[26] Prolonged grief around decline in health or physical functioning may be associated with greater use of health care services (eg, emergency room visits, hospitalizations).[27] Further, up to 25% of older adults who have experienced a major bereavement may go on to experience complicated grief, which refers specifically to an atypical, maladaptive, and prolonged grief reaction.[28–30] The boundary between what is normal after a loss and what constitutes a disorder is a topic of debate, including regarding the recent change in the fifth version of the DSM released in 2013.[9] In this version, a controversial change was made to remove an exclusion for a major depressive episode for bereavement, which in previous DSM versions had ruled out a diagnosis of major depressive disorder for individuals within 2 months after bereavement except in severe cases.[31] Although there are several arguments both in support and opposition of this change,[31] the implication for clinicians is the critical need to use best judgment in distinguishing a normative grief reaction from complicated grief or a depressive syndrome. Some of the research to date on differences between normal or uncomplicated grief, complicated grief, and depression or anxiety may be useful in making diagnostic decisions.

Common predictors for a greater risk of complicated grief across studies are female gender, older age, lower education, and poorer cognitive functioning.[28,29,32] Anticipation or expectancy around the loss (ie, whether an older widow expected the death of her spouse to occur) has not been shown to be predictive of differences in grief.[33] Among those with complicated grief, up to 10% may experience comorbid depression and 17% comorbid anxiety.[29] Of note, the emotional responses to bereavement may mitigate across time; for example, in 1 study, differences in depressive symptoms and psychopathology between widowed older adults and nonwidowed older adults that had been evident 2 months after a loss faded to nonsignificance within 12 months, although differences in grief-specific symptoms remained to some extent even up to 2.5 years after the loss.[34] Given that the DSM's bereavement exception extended only to 2 months after a loss, these results highlight the more protracted trajectory that recovery from grief and its emotional associates may take.

Research indicates that there is not a consistent, clear definition and boundary between complicated grief and uncomplicated or normal grief and, throughout the literature, symptoms of complicated grief and depression or anxiety significantly overlap.[30] Also, a comprehensive framework of bereavement and grief must take into account pre-loss factors (eg, preexisting depression), interpersonal and intrapersonal factors (eg, social support, physical health and functioning), and cognitive coping (eg, cognitive appraisal, emotion regulation), all of which influence grief outcomes and resilience.[30] Finally, cultural sensitivity to grief and mourning-related norms and practices is critical, although little is currently known about cultural differences in this area.[30]

Grief may present in many heterogeneous ways among older adults who have experienced bereavement and has the potential to impact risk for depression and anxiety. Clinicians should use their best judgment to distinguish normative grief responses, complicated grief, and depression or anxiety syndromes. Preloss functioning, as well as current functioning and the individual's trajectory of change in grief symptoms over time, may help to distinguish these phenomena.

SOCIAL ISOLATION AND LONELINESS

Aging is associated with changes in the size and composition of social networks, such that, as we age, the size of our social networks tends to decrease, with decreases primarily seen regarding friends and other nonfamily connections.[1] This finding was originally attributed to the many losses that occur in later life, including retirement (and loss of work relationships), declining health, and deaths of friends and family. However, gerontologists have documented that the decreased size of social networks associated with aging is actually due, in large part, to an active process by older adults to "prune" their networks and discard the less meaningful and valued ties to devote more energy and time to the most meaningful relationships.[1] Thus, although social networks tend to be smaller in later life, older adults report greater satisfaction with their social networks. Further, although loneliness and social isolation are often described as a problem of old age in the popular media, loneliness and social isolation are not the norm in later life. In fact, a recent study with a large sample representative of the US population found that the prevalence of loneliness decreases with age.[35] In contrast, up to one-third of community-dwelling older adults report that they expect to become lonely as they grow older or that they agree with the statement, "old age is a time of loneliness."[36] In turn, those who agree with these stereotypes of aging are then more likely to actually experience loneliness in the future, consistent with a "self-fulfilling prophecy."[36] Addressing expectations about aging to be more positive and realistic can be a useful intervention for individuals at all ages, patients, caregivers, and clinicians.

This is not to say that social isolation and loneliness are not relevant issues for older adults. Although social isolation and loneliness are not the norm in later life, when they do occur, they may have even more deleterious effects on health and well-being than at younger ages owing to the body's decreased capacity for managing stress (cf., the strength and vulnerability integration theory discussed in the Introduction). Further, social isolation and loneliness may be key targets of intervention to promote health and well-being in later life because these aspects of our social health remain malleable throughout our lives, whereas some factors, such as sensory impairment or loss of mobility may be less amenable to intervention. Thus, promoting social connectedness and social well-being is a promising intervention strategy in later life. However, the research literature on *how* to promote social connectedness and decrease loneliness is in its infancy for individuals at any age.[37] What is known, however, suggests that, to effectively help an older patient with isolation and/or loneliness, it is useful to understand the context in which these experiences are occurring and what the older adult believes is the primary cause. Research with older adults has confirmed that loneliness is due in part to objective circumstances—increasing disability and frailty, environmental barriers to socialization, and bereavement, whereas other research emphasizes the role of subjective perceptions, such as thinking of oneself as useless, in causing and perpetuating loneliness.[38,39] Each of these potential contributors to loneliness and isolation can be addressed through various interventions, such as care management to address transportation barriers, hearing aids to promote communication, psychotherapy to promote motivation to engage, and access to meaningful social activities, such as volunteering or educational opportunities.

For older adults with moderate to advanced dementia, or other illnesses that impact the ability to understand and communicate one's needs, a lack of social stimulation and loneliness can be one contributor to agitation or aggressive behavior that is distressing to both the patient and caregivers. These types of behaviors that are considered abnormal and problematic can sometimes occur when an older person is not able to communicate a very normal and healthy need, such as social connections and comfort. All humans have an innate need to belong to social relationships and groups.[40] When this need is not met, loneliness and distress emerges at all ages. When working with older adults who may be demonstrating abnormal behaviors, it is useful to consider whether a normal and healthy unmet need is contributing to the behavior.

SUICIDAL IDEATION AND BEHAVIOR

Older adults, specifically older men, have the highest rates of suicide in the United States[3] and around the world,[4] with risk increasing with age through late life. In the United States, white men aged 85 and older have the highest rates of suicide deaths, almost four times the rate in the general population (ie, 47.17 per 100,000 vs 14.21 per 100,000).[3] Among older Americans who reported suicidal ideation in the past year, 12.7% reported at least 1 suicide attempt in the past year.[41] Older adults who attempt suicide are known to be at exponentially greater risk for death, although exact statistics are difficult to find; some estimates state that whereas there are 25 attempts for every suicide death nationally within the United States, among older adults there are only 4 attempts to every suicide death,[42] therefore making nonlethal suicide attempts less common. Therefore, it is critically important to identify suicidal ideation and risk early in this age group, before it escalates into an attempt. Risk factors for suicide among older adults include the "5 Ds": depression and other psychiatric illnesses, disease (physical illness), disability (pain and functional impairment), social disconnectedness, and access to deadly means (such as firearms).[43,44]

Given the importance of identifying suicidal ideation early, understanding the difference between normative thoughts or attitudes about death in late life and maladaptive thoughts that could contribute to risk for suicide is critical. Older adults do demonstrate differences in their attitudes and reactions toward death compared with younger and middle-aged adults, such that they report overall less fear of death and greater acceptance of death,[45] and exhibit less attentional avoidance to death-related information.[46,47] Acceptance of death can be a neutral view of death as natural and inevitable, or even a positive view of death as a gateway to a positive afterlife. However, a lesser fear of death and greater acceptance of death with a particular focus on escaping negative situations or experiences in life are associated with a wish to die.[48] Passive suicidal ideation—going beyond just acceptance of death—refers to thoughts of being better off dead, or a desire to die, without specific thoughts of ending one's own life. (Active) suicidal ideation—refers to thoughts of ending one's own life. One study estimated that 10% to 13% of all adults age 50 and older experience passive suicidal ideation.[49] Despite misconceptions that passive suicidal ideation is less concerning than active suicidal ideation, or even normal among older adults, studies have shown that even passive suicidal ideation is associated with an increased risk for suicidal behavior and should not be considered normative.[50,51] Further, some research has shown that individuals may transition between passive and active suicidal ideation in a given episode.[52] The studies reviewed here suggest that, although older adults may exhibit less avoidance of death-related topics and greater overall acceptance of death, it is problematic when older adults express a desire for their life to end, even without active thoughts of ending one's own life.

Assessment of suicide risk by health care providers is essential, because many older adults who die by suicide have had recent contact with a health care provider, but may not have contact with any mental health provider. More than three-quarters (77%) of adults age 55 and older who die by suicide have had contact with a primary care physician within the past year, with 58% having contact within the past month, compared with 8.5% in the past year and 11.0% in the past month having contact with mental health care.[53] Almost one-third (29%) of adults age 50 and older who die by suicide have contact with a primary health care provider within 1 week of their death.[54] However, general medical providers may be less likely to screen for suicidal ideation and risk and implement important interventions. Among Veterans Affairs patients who attempted suicide, older adults' charts were less likely to show documentation by general medical providers of assessment for certain risk factors for suicide (eg, access to firearms) or interventions to reduce suicide risk (eg, safety planning, mental health care referrals) compared with younger adults.[19]

Although assessment for suicidality should occur for all patients with depression, suicidal ideation can also occur among those without depression, and therefore it is important to use best judgment in screening for suicide risk in a primary care or other medical population.[55,56] Although a clinician may use an assessment instrument to screen for suicidal ideation, such as the Patient Health Questionnaire-9, it is important to follow-up with specific questions about types of suicidal thoughts, plans, access to means, intent, and so on.[55,56] The P4 Screener may be a useful tool, because it was designed as a brief follow-up to the Patient Health Questionnaire-9.[57] Also, relying on assessments of depression may miss older adults who have suicidal ideation but are not reporting symptoms of depression.[55] It is important to have mental health care, implemented within an effective referral and transfer of care system, available for those who do exhibit an increased risk for suicide.[55,56] In addition to referrals to more intensive mental health care, brief interventions such as safety planning[58] may be implemented within medical clinics and emergency departments.

DISCUSSION AND SUMMARY

A common misconception, likely rooted in ageist societal biases, is that emotional turmoil or negative affective experiences are the norm in later life[6–8]; lifespan theory and research demonstrates that this is not true, and can negatively impact diagnosis and treatment by providers as well as expectations and physical and mental health outcomes in patients themselves.[7,8] However, in certain contexts older adults may be vulnerable to experiencing grief, social isolation, and/or loneliness and have a heightened risk of suicide. Although older adults experience greater psychological resilience to negative affect, they also experience age-related physiologic vulnerabilities.[14] **Fig. 1** illustrates the risk and resilience factors for affective well-being commonly experienced in late life, as discussed throughout this review, as weights on a balance scale. Although the majority of older adults benefit in late life from greater positive affect via flexible coping and decreased reactivity to negative affect, as well as

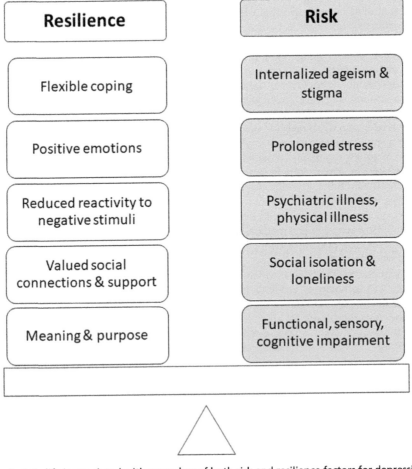

Fig. 1. Late life is associated with a number of both risk and resilience factors for depression and anxiety. Although older adulthood is generally a time of positive affective well-being owing to resilience factors pictured, the presence of the outlined risk factors may contribute to negative affective outcomes.

more meaningful and valued social connections, those who experience prolonged stressors, physiologic risk factors such as illness or impairment and decreased physiologic resilience to stress, as well as social isolation or loneliness, along with internalized ageist views of late life may be at elevated risk for depression, anxiety, or other negative outcomes. Viewing risk and resilience factors this way highlights the usefulness of considering the combination of factors (eg, if multiple risk factors are "piling up" for a given patient, in the absence of some resilience factors) rather than assessing each factor in isolation. Additionally, strengthening protective factors, even when risk factors are currently minimal, can serve as a valuable prevention tool against future risks.

Affective problems such as depression and anxiety may be more difficult to diagnose in older adults, owing to unclear differentiation between normative experiences (eg, bereavement and uncomplicated grief) and maladaptive syndromes (eg, complicated grief), differences in symptom presentation in this age group, and comorbid physical and cognitive conditions. It is critical for those working with older adults to use criteria and assessment instruments that are tailored to the unique needs and presentations of older adults, rather than depending on criteria and instruments that do not reflect this age group. The most important factor in determining diagnosis and the need for treatment is the impact on the individual's everyday functioning. If treatment is needed, implementation of or referral for appropriate treatments that are evidence based in older adults (eg, cognitive behavioral therapy,[59] problem solving therapy,[59,60] antidepressant treatment[61]) may significantly improve mood and quality of life.

CLINICS CARE POINTS

- Use of criteria and assessment instruments validated in older adults is necessary. The Geriatric Depression Scale (https://consultgeri.org/try-this/general-assessment/issue-4.pdf) and Geriatric Anxiety Inventory are examples of such instruments.
- The Patient Health Questionnaire-9 and P4 screener (https://gerocentral.org/wp-content/uploads/2013/04/P4-Suicide-Risk-Screener.pdf), in conjunction with a detailed clinical interview, may be used to assess risk for suicide.
- Safety planning (https://www.mirecc.va.gov/visn16/collaborative-safety-planning-manual.asp) is a brief, effective intervention that can help to manage suicide risk in a clinical setting.

DISCLOSURE

The authors have nothing to disclose. This work was supported by an NIMH National Research Service Award Postdoctoral Fellowship (T32MH20061; Conwell, PI).

REFERENCES

1. Charles ST, Carstensen LL. Social and emotional aging. Annu Rev Psychol 2010; 61:383–409.
2. Fiske A, Wetherell JL, Gatz M. Depression in older adults. Annu Rev Clin Psychol 2009;5:363–89.
3. Centers for Disease Control and Prevention NCfIPaC. Web-based Injury Statistics Query and Reporting System (WISQARS). 2019. Available at: https://www.cdc.gov/injury/wisqars/index.html. Accessed June 22, 2020.

4. World Health Organization. Preventing suicide: a global imperative. Geneva (Switzerland): World Health Organization; 2014.

5. Wuthrich VM, Johnco CJ, Wetherell JL. Differences in anxiety and depression symptoms: comparison between older and younger clinical samples. Int Psychogeriatr 2015;27(9):1523–32.

6. Haigh EAP, Bogucki OE, Sigmon ST, et al. Depression among older adults: a 20-year update on five common myths and misconceptions. Am J Geriatr Psychiatry 2018;26(1):107–22.

7. Uncapher H, Arean PA. Physicians are less willing to treat suicidal ideation in older patients. J Am Geriatr Soc 2000;48(2):188–92.

8. Nelson TD. Promoting healthy aging by confronting ageism. Am Psychol 2016; 71(4):276–82.

9. American Psychiatric Association. Diagnostic and statistical manual of mental disorders. 5th edition. Arlington (VA): American Psychiatric Association; 2013.

10. World Health Organization. The ICD-10 classification of mental and behavioural disorders: clinical descriptions and diagnostic guidelines. Geneva (Switzerland): World Health Organization; 1992.

11. Carstensen LL, Turan B, Scheibe S, et al. Emotional experience improves with age: evidence based on over 10 years of experience sampling. Psychol Aging 2011;26(1):21–33.

12. Carstensen LL, Isaacowitz DM, Charles ST. Taking time seriously. A theory of socioemotional selectivity. Am Psychol 1999;54(3):165–81.

13. Charles ST. Strength and vulnerability integration: a model of emotional well-being across adulthood. Psychol Bull 2010;136(6):1068–91.

14. Mather M. The emotion paradox in the aging brain. Ann N Y Acad Sci 2012; 1251(1):33–49.

15. Gonzalez HM, Tarraf W, Whitfield KE, et al. The epidemiology of major depression and ethnicity in the United States. J Psychiatr Res 2010;44(15):1043–51.

16. Mackenzie CS, El-Gabalawy R, Chou KL, et al. Prevalence and predictors of persistent versus remitting mood, anxiety, and substance disorders in a national sample of older adults. Am J Geriatr Psychiatry 2014;22(9):854–65.

17. Byers AL, Yaffe K, Covinsky KE, et al. High occurrence of mood and anxiety disorders among older adults: The National Comorbidity Survey Replication. Arch Gen Psychiatry 2010;67(5):489–96.

18. Bryant C. Anxiety and depression in old age: challenges in recognition and diagnosis. Int Psychogeriatr 2010;22(4):511–3.

19. Simons K, Van Orden K, Conner KR, et al. Age differences in suicide risk screening and management prior to suicide attempts. Am J Geriatr Psychiatry 2019;27(6):604–8.

20. Hegeman JM, Kok RM, van der Mast RC, et al. Phenomenology of depression in older compared with younger adults: meta-analysis. Br J Psychiatry 2012;200(4): 275–81.

21. Laborde-Lahoz P, El-Gabalawy R, Kinley J, et al. Subsyndromal depression among older adults in the USA: prevalence, comorbidity, and risk for new-onset psychiatric disorders in late life. Int J Geriatr Psychiatry 2015;30(7):677–85.

22. Gould CE, Gerolimatos LA, Beaudreau SA, et al. Older adults report more sadness and less jealousy than young adults in response to worry induction. Aging Ment Health 2018;22(4):512–8.

23. Mohlman J, Bryant C, Lenze EJ, et al. Improving recognition of late life anxiety disorders in Diagnostic and Statistical Manual of Mental Disorders, Fifth Edition:

observations and recommendations of the Advisory Committee to the Lifespan Disorders Work Group. Int J Geriatr Psychiatry 2012;27(6):549–56.

24. Yesavage JA, Brink TL, Rose TL, et al. Development and validation of a geriatric depression screening scale: a preliminary report. J Psychiatr Res 1983;17(1):37–49.

25. Pachana NA, Byrne GJ, Siddle H, et al. Development and validation of the geriatric anxiety inventory. Int Psychogeriatr 2007;19(1):103–14.

26. Shear MK, Ghesquiere A, Glickman K. Bereavement and complicated grief. Curr Psychiatry Rep 2013;15(11):406.

27. Holland JM, Graves S, Klingspon KL, et al. Prolonged grief symptoms related to loss of physical functioning: examining unique associations with medical service utilization. Disabil Rehabil 2016;38(3):205–10.

28. Kersting A, Brahler E, Glaesmer H, et al. Prevalence of complicated grief in a representative population-based sample. J Affect Disord 2011;131(1–3):339–43.

29. Newson RS, Boelen PA, Hek K, et al. The prevalence and characteristics of complicated grief in older adults. J Affect Disord 2011;132(1–2):231–8.

30. Shah SN, Meeks S. Late-life bereavement and complicated grief: a proposed comprehensive framework. Aging Ment Health 2012;16(1):39–56.

31. Iglewicz A, Seay K, Zetumer SD, et al. The removal of the bereavement exclusion in the DSM-5: exploring the evidence. Curr Psychiatry Rep 2013;15(11):413.

32. Nielsen MK, Carlsen AH, Neergaard MA, et al. Looking beyond the mean in grief trajectories: a prospective, population-based cohort study. Soc Sci Med 2019;232:460–9.

33. Dessonville C, Thompson LW, Gallagher D. The role of anticipatory bereavement in older women's adjustment to widowhood. Gerontologist 1988;28(6):792–6.

34. Thompson LW, Gallagher-Thompson D, Futterman A, et al. The effects of late-life spousal bereavement over a 30-month interval. Psychol Aging 1991;6(3):434–41.

35. Bruce LD, Wu JS, Lustig SL, et al. Loneliness in the United States: a 2018 national panel survey of demographic, structural, cognitive, and behavioral characteristics. Am J Health Promot 2019;33(8):1123–33.

36. Pikhartova J, Bowling A, Victor C. Is loneliness in later life a self-fulfilling prophecy? Aging Ment Health 2016;20(5):543–9.

37. Dickens AP, Richards SH, Greaves CJ, et al. Interventions targeting social isolation in older people: a systematic review. BMC Public Health 2011;11:647.

38. Qualter P, Vanhalst J, Harris R, et al. Loneliness across the life span. Perspect Psychol Sci 2015;10(2):250–64.

39. Cacioppo JT, Cacioppo S, Boomsma DI. Evolutionary mechanisms for loneliness. Cogn Emot 2014;28(1):3–21.

40. Baumeister RF, Leary MR. The need to belong: desire for interpersonal attachments as a fundamental human motivation. Psychol Bull 1995;117(3):497–529.

41. Han B, Compton WM, Gfroerer J, et al. Prevalence and correlates of past 12-month suicide attempt among adults with past-year suicidal ideation in the United States. J Clin Psychiatry 2015;76(3):295–302.

42. Drapeau CW, McIntosh JL. U.S.A. suicide 2017: official final data. Washington, DC: American Association of Suicidology; 2018.

43. Van Orden K, Conwell Y. Suicides in late life. Curr Psychiatry Rep 2011;13(3):234–41.

44. Conwell Y. Suicide and suicide prevention in later life. Focus 2013;11(1):39–47.

45. Gesser G, Wong PTP, Reker GT. Death attitudes across the life-span: the development and validation of the death attitude profile (DAP). OMEGA - Journal of Death and Dying 1988;18(2):113–28.

46. De Raedt R, Koster EH, Ryckewaert R. Aging and attentional bias for death related and general threat-related information: less avoidance in older as compared with middle-aged adults. J Gerontol B Psychol Sci Soc Sci 2013; 68(1):41–8.

47. Maxfield M, Pyszczynski T, Kluck B, et al. Age-related differences in responses to thoughts of one's own death: mortality salience and judgments of moral transgressions. Psychol Aging 2007;22(2):341–53.

48. Bonnewyn A, Shah A, Bruffaerts R, et al. Are religiousness and death attitudes associated with the wish to die in older people? Int Psychogeriatr 2016;28(3): 397–404.

49. Dong L, Kalesnikava VA, Gonzalez R, et al. Beyond depression: estimating 12-months prevalence of passive suicidal ideation in mid- and late-life in the health and retirement study. Am J Geriatr Psychiatry 2019;27(12):1399–410.

50. Van Orden KA, O'Riley AA, Simning A, et al. Passive suicide ideation: an indicator of risk among older adults seeking aging services? Gerontologist 2015;55(6): 972–80.

51. Van Orden KA, Simning A, Conwell Y, et al. Characteristics and comorbid symptoms of older adults reporting death ideation. Am J Geriatr Psychiatry 2013;21(8): 803–10.

52. Szanto K, Reynolds CF 3rd, Frank E, et al. Suicide in elderly depressed patients: is active vs. passive suicidal ideation a clinically valid distinction? Am J Geriatr Psychiatry 1996;4:197–207.

53. Luoma JB, Martin CE, Pearson JL. Contact with mental health and primary care providers before suicide: a review of the evidence. Am J Psychiatry 2002;159: 909–16.

54. Stene-Larsen K, Reneflot A. Contact with primary and mental health care prior to suicide: a systematic review of the literature from 2000 to 2017. Scand J Public Health 2019;47(1):9–17.

55. Raue PJ, Ghesquiere AR, Bruce ML. Suicide risk in primary care: identification and management in older adults. Curr Psychiatry Rep 2014;16(9):466.

56. McDowell AK, Lineberry TW, Bostwick JM. Practical suicide-risk management for the busy primary care physician. Mayo Clin Proc 2011;86(8):792–800.

57. Dube P, Kurt K, Bair MJ, et al. The p4 screener: evaluation of a brief measure for assessing potential suicide risk in 2 randomized effectiveness trials of primary care and oncology patients. Prim Care Companion J Clin Psychiatry 2010; 12(6):PCC.

58. Conti EC, Jahn DR, Simons KV, et al. Safety planning to manage suicide risk with older adults: case examples and recommendations. Clin Gerontol 2020;43(1): 104–9.

59. Renn BN, Arean PA. Psychosocial treatment options for major depressive disorder in older adults. Curr Treat Options Psychiatry 2017;4(1):1–12.

60. Kirkham JG, Choi N, Seitz DP. Meta-analysis of problem solving therapy for the treatment of major depressive disorder in older adults. Int J Geriatr Psychiatry 2016;31(5):526–35.

61. Kok RM, Reynolds CF 3rd. Management of depression in older adults: a review. JAMA 2017;317(20):2114–22.

Musculoskeletal Pain in Older Adults: A Clinical Review

Travis P. Welsh, MD[a], Ailing E. Yang, BA[a],
Una E. Makris, MD, MSc[a,b],*

KEYWORDS

- Persistent pain • Multidisciplinary • Aging • Nonpharmacologic • Musculoskeletal

KEY POINTS

- Musculoskeletal pain in older adults contributes to physical disability and impairments in psychosocial domains of health including social isolation, depression, and anxiety.
- The manifestations of persistent pain in older adults are frequently a result of multiple contributing factors.
- A comprehensive musculoskeletal pain assessment includes pain location, intensity, interference with daily life, and pain-related behaviors with attention given to how these affect and interact with comorbidities, function, mood, and cognition.
- A wide array of nonpharmacologic and pharmacologic therapies exists for the treatment of persistent pain, and they can be tailored to the patient's specific comorbidities, functional ability, preferences, and treatment goals.
- Because of the inherent complexity of musculoskeletal pain in older adults, management should be multidisciplinary, multimodal, and emphasize a strong therapeutic alliance while addressing domains of pain, functionality, mental health, and social engagement.

INTRODUCTION/BACKGROUND

Among older adults, persistent musculoskeletal pain is highly prevalent, with rates ranging from 40% to 60%.[1] Multisite pain contributes to significant disability among older adults.[2] Persistent pain is defined as pain that extends beyond the usual period of healing, typically for longer than 3 to 6 months. Musculoskeletal disorders are recognized as a significant threat to maintaining health in older age[3] and have been associated with falls, frailty, depression, anxiety, sleep disturbance, reduced mobility,

[a] Department of Internal Medicine, UT Southwestern Medical Center, Dallas, TX, USA;
[b] Medical Service, VA North Texas Health Care System, Dallas, TX, USA
* Corresponding author. Department of Internal Medicine, Division of Rheumatic Diseases, UT Southwestern Medical Center, VA North Texas Health Care System, 5323 Harry Hines Boulevard, Dallas, TX 75390-9169.
E-mail addresses: una.makris@utsouthwestern.edu; una.makris2@va.gov
Twitter: @AilingEYang (A.E.Y.); @UnaMakris (U.E.M.)

Med Clin N Am 104 (2020) 855–872
https://doi.org/10.1016/j.mcna.2020.05.002
0025-7125/20/© 2020 Elsevier Inc. All rights reserved.

and impaired cognitive function.[4-8] Additionally, medical treatments for pain have been estimated to cost the United States about $300 billion annually, and this burden continues to increase.[9] Unfortunately, pain may be undertreated or inappropriately managed in older adults for several reasons, including lack of identification of pain, false belief that pain is part of the aging process, cognitive impairment with variable pain presentations, patient underreporting, and limited time in clinical practice to address pain among multiple comorbid conditions.[10,11] This highlights the importance of understanding the special considerations in the assessment and management of persistent musculoskeletal pain in older adults.

Persistent pain should be considered in the context of geriatric syndromes. For example, falls, frailty, cognitive decline/dementia, and sleep disturbance are often linked to persistent pain.[12] Studies have shown a relationship between moderate to severe pain and accelerated memory decline and impairments in attention and executive function in community-dwelling older adults.[8,13] Given the multitude of contributing factors and its close relationship with geriatric syndromes, persistent pain in older adults is regarded by some experts as a geriatric syndrome.[14]

Older adults are particularly prone to living with multiple illnesses, which affects treatment considerations. Defined as the presence of more than two comorbid conditions, multimorbidity is estimated to exist in at least half the geriatric population.[15] Consequently, polypharmacy, often described as being prescribed five medications or more, is also common; it has been linked with falls, increased mortality, and longer hospital stays.[16] This highlights the need for careful review of relative risks and benefits of medications in older adults when treating pain, because the unintended adverse effects on comorbid conditions, and polypharmacy could nullify potential benefits of another added medication.

Mental health should be carefully considered in the context of pain. The relationship between persistent pain and depression and anxiety is well-established and complex, with contributions including augmentation of functional impairment, neuroinflammatory changes, impaired social engagement, and maladaptive coping.[17,18] Furthermore, there seems to be a reciprocal relationship between pain and depression in older adults, with pain and depression being independent risk factors for one another.[19] This association underscores the complexity of the pain experience in older adults and re-emphasizes a comprehensive biopsychosocial approach to managing persistent pain.

Within a comprehensive approach, the clinician should consider the age-related changes in organ function that have significant impact on the pharmacodynamics and pharmacokinetics of medications.[20] Normal age-related decline in renal and liver function may affect drug processing, reducing clearance rates and changing efficacy. Decreased muscle mass and increased adiposity can also affect the volume of distribution of medications in older adults, affecting tolerability and efficacy of medications. These changes emphasize the importance of avoiding a "one size fits all" approach when prescribing medications to older adults.

Patients have unique pain experiences, which are heavily influenced by the type of pain, physical perception of pain, emotional state and reaction to pain, ability to cope with pain, and the patient's personal beliefs about pain. When approaching persistent pain in older adults, it is critical to engage in collaborative care to assess and address these multiple unique contributing factors. In this review, we encourage a comprehensive assessment followed by a multidisciplinary approach to pain management that emphasizes rehabilitation and nonpharmacologic modalities, particularly appropriate for complex older adults.

GENERAL APPROACH
Assessment: History

The assessment of pain in older adults begins with obtaining a complete history that characterizes the type of pain and then further quantifies the impact the pain has on function, interference with daily activities, pain-related behaviors, and effect on psychological and social well-being. Older adults may have differing perspectives and beliefs about pain as compared with younger adults, which may affect pain reporting. Stoicism and potential fear or embarrassment about pain may contribute to underreporting of pain in this patient group.[21,22] A comprehensive evaluation that includes all dimensions of the pain experience is the first step to effectively manage pain, because this information guides treatment.

The ideal source of pain history is the patient (self-report). However, for patients with cognitive impairment, dementia, and limited ability to communicate about pain, obtaining an accurate firsthand account of pain may not be feasible. As a result, several observer-based pain scales incorporate pain-based behaviors of facial response, vocalization, or body posture to characterize the pain being experienced by the patient according to level of cognitive ability.[23] These tools, however, have variable interrater reliability and test-retest reliability.[24] Obtaining collateral information from loved ones and caregivers (proxy-reports) is beneficial. Proxy-reporting is useful to help identify, characterize, and monitor pain for patients who are not able to communicate their pain symptoms.

Characterization of pain should include specific locations, quality, aggravating or relieving factors, and time course. With consideration of nociceptive, neuropathic, or central sensitization of pain, identification of cause when possible is useful for tailoring medical treatments, although sometimes a definitive cause cannot be identified. More than one cause may be present. Prior trials of treatments often dictate what a patient is willing to try next; therefore, clinicians should document how previous pharmacologic therapies, nonpharmacologic therapies, and prior pain-related surgeries were or were not effective. Similarly, understanding the pain in the context of other medical conditions, and how the patient prioritizes the importance of these, is also critical when deciding on a management plan. A comprehensive approach to assessment of chronic low back pain (cLBP) is found in several publications of the 2014 "Report of the Task Force on Research Standards for Chronic Low Back Pain," where musculoskeletal pain experts and leaders convened to recommend a minimal dataset to help guide clinicians and researchers on important domains to measure when managing persistent pain.[25] Using this minimal dataset as an outline, **Box 1** provides a list of appropriate domains to assess for chronic musculoskeletal pain in older adults.

An important and often overlooked portion of the comprehensive pain assessment is understanding the patient's expectations for what defines therapeutic success. The history facilitates this conversation, because understanding the daily impact of pain often can help identify specific areas of pain the patient would like to focus on. Although "pain-free" may not be a realistic goal, it is likely that with multimodal approaches, the patient will be able to manage the pain and associated symptoms while improving function. Anchoring conversations about pain management in patient-identified values and realistic goals of care is central, because individual-specific experiences, such as engagement in social activities, ability to enjoy favorite hobbies, and more restful sleep, all contribute to the pain experience.

Box 1
Domains relevant for assessing chronic musculoskeletal pain in older adults

Location of pain

Duration of pain (in months and years)

Characterization of pain: acute, subacute, chronic

Frequency and interference of pain
• Pain intensity with numerical rating scale, based on recall from past 7 days

Referred pain or radicular symptoms

Other sites of pain: gastrointestinal, headaches, widespread, etc

Prior surgeries: type, date, response

Prior treatment modalities used for pain management
• Lifestyle changes
• Psychological/behavioral
• Physical therapy and rehabilitation
• Complementary, alternative, and mind-body approaches
• Pharmacotherapy

Physical function: doing chores (eg, vacuuming, yard work), climbing stairs, walking for at least 15 minutes, running errands

Mental health: depression, anxiety, post-traumatic stress disorder (as appropriate)

Sleep disturbance

Alcohol use

Tobacco use

Demographics: age, gender, race/ethnicity, employment status, highest educational attainment, body mass index

These domains and categories were adapted based on the Minimal Dataset from the 2014 Report of the NIH Task Force on Research Standards for Chronic Low Back Pain.

Adapted from Deyo RA, Dworkin SF, Amtmann D, et al. Report of the NIH Task Force on Research Standards for Chronic Low Back Pain. *J Pain.* 2014;15(6):569-585; with permission.

Physical Examination

The physical examination for persistent pain includes visual inspection, palpation of painful sites, and quantification of strength and range of motion of the affected painful areas. When applicable, the clinician should also examine the joint contralateral to the affected joint to assess for symmetric joint involvement. Joints proximal and distal to the site of pain should be examined, specifically considering sources of referred pain, such as in the presentation of knee pain presenting with contributing hip, iliotibial band, and/or ankle pathology. Gait should be assessed for abnormalities, which can hint at underlying core issues, such as deficiencies in strength, sensation, or coordination. The Timed Up and Go Test is an efficient and valuable tool to evaluate mobility and is often used as part of a frailty assessment.[26] Examination of the patient's behaviors and reactions to elicited pain are especially useful for those with cognitive impairment, because it can help to better stratify pain intensity. Outside of these core principles, the provider should tailor the examination with location-specific maneuvers.

Imaging

Abnormal imaging findings are common in older adults. Such findings as degenerative changes of the spine or hips do not necessarily contribute meaningfully to the assessment of pain or disability. The key to interpreting imaging for musculoskeletal pain is determining whether the clinical picture correlates with the findings seen on imaging. Plain film radiography can help to assess degree of joint degeneration or investigate for other possible cause of symptoms. Findings often do not reliably correlate with pain frequency or intensity, and use of imaging often does not lead to improved outcomes.[27] Because of its frequently limited utility, imaging can put unnecessary extra psychological and financial burden on a patient.[28] Imaging should be considered on a case-by-case basis, especially when "red-flag" symptoms suggest an urgent issue to be assessed.

MANAGEMENT APPROACHES
The Team

The management of persistent pain in the older adult involves multiple modalities (non-pharmacologic, rehabilitative, pharmacologic, and possibly surgical) as depicted in **Fig. 1**. Therefore, it is important to enlist the help of a diverse team to address the various domains of pain and related comorbidities, also listed in **Fig. 1**. Naturally, if an older patient has multiple comorbid conditions, the number of subspecialists can become overwhelming. Clear communication, especially in large teams, is key. Each member of the team is vitally important and builds the therapeutic relationship with the patient. Counseling on the expected course of persistent pain and providing reassurance are keys to progress in therapy.

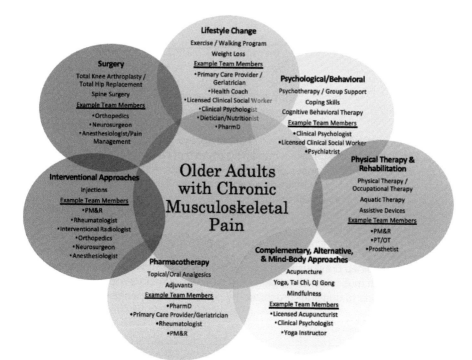

Fig. 1. Components of multimodal interdisciplinary management of older adults with chronic musculoskeletal pain. PM&R, physical medicine and rehabilitation; PT/OT, physical therapists/occupational therapists.

Nonpharmacologic Modalities: First-Line

A comprehensive and effective treatment regimen uses multiple modalities for treatment with preference for nonpharmacologic therapies. Although these are considered first-line therapies in guidelines,[29] they are unfortunately often offered after multiple trials of pharmacologic therapies and more invasive modalities. Nonpharmacologic therapies are particularly attractive for use in older adults because of the ratio of effectiveness versus safety. Nonpharmacologic modalities include physical therapy, occupational therapy, exercise (including walking) programs, psychological interventions (cognitive behavioral therapy, acceptance, pain coping skills training, cognitive restructuring, and commitment therapy),[30] and complementary, alternative, and mind-body approaches and are tailored to a patient's explicit abilities, preferences, and goals of treatment. Physical activity is consistently recommended to be a key component of any treatment plan for persistent pain in older adults.[28,29,31] Exercise can reduce mortality, improve function, increase strength, reduce risk of cardiovascular disease, promote social interaction, and relieve pain. It has also been shown that providing specific physical activity advice, a plan of action, and a plan for follow-up are important in uptake and maintenance of an exercise program in older adults.[32] In many patients, behavioral and psychological interventions for persistent pain are effective. For example, mindfulness programs have short- and long-term pain reduction and short-term functional improvements.[33] Mindfulness and meditation therapies hold promise for improvements in pain and function, although more studies are needed to better understand their effect.[34] These interventions should be considered in the context of feasibility, availability, access, cost, and patient motivation to participate.

Pharmacologic Options

When considering pharmacologic therapies, the mantra is often "start low and go slow," titrating medications while observing for adverse effects. **Table 1** outlines the classes of medications typically used in the management of persistent pain in older adults. Sometimes, an augmented pain-relieving effect is achieved when combining medications from two different drug classes. Opioids are not recommended in guidelines for managing osteoarthritis (OA). As mentioned, one must carefully consider the comorbidities and risks associated with each selected medication.

Regular follow-up is critical when managing persistent pain in older adults.[29] Follow-up visits assess for effectiveness of the management approach, provide an opportunity for encouragement to sustain pain-reducing behavioral changes, and allow for monitoring of adverse effects of treatments. These visits can also serve to build trust and strengthen the therapeutic alliance between the patient and provider.

COMMON MUSCULOSKELETAL CONDITIONS IN OLDER ADULTS

The principles outlined previously are a general approach to assessment and management of persistent musculoskeletal pain in older adults. The next sections outline specific considerations to consider organized by common musculoskeletal conditions in older adults.

Osteoarthritis

OA is the most common type of arthritis, and about half of all adults older than the age of 65 in the United States have doctor-diagnosed OA.[39] Age is one of the strongest risk factors for OA, with others being gender (women have higher rates and report more severe symptoms), overweight/obesity, joint misalignment (varus or valgus deformity),

Table 1
Common pharmacologic approaches for older adults with musculoskeletal pain

Treatment	Indications	Safety Considerations	Recent Guidelines
Topical agents			
Capsaicin	Minor muscle/joint pain (backache, strains, sprains, arthritis, bruises, cramps, muscle stiffness or soreness); neuropathic pain associated with diabetic neuropathy or postherpetic neuralgia	Wash hands with soap and water immediately after applying (unless hands are part of the treatment area) or apply with gloves Do not use within 1 h before a bath or immediately after a bath Avoid concurrent use with other topical agents or heating pad	Conditionally recommended for knee OA Conditionally recommended against hand OA Insufficient data on hip OA[35]
Methyl salicylate and menthol	Minor muscle/joint pain and aches (backache, strains, sprains, arthritis, bruises)	Do not apply to face, wounds, rashes, damaged skin, mucous membranes, or immediately after a bath Avoid concurrent use with other topical agents or heating pad	Apply patch for up to 8 h (max: 2 patches/24 h)
Lidocaine	Postherpetic neuralgia, minor localized pain	Use lowest effective dose for pain relief for shortest duration of time (prolonged exposure increases risk for systemic absorption, potentially leading to CNS and cardiac effects) Avoid contact with water or external heat sources	Insufficient data in OA Apply patch for up to 12 h (max: 1 patch/24 h)
NSAIDs	Osteoarthritis in knee and hand; may also be used for ankle, elbow, foot, or wrist; acute pain (strains, sprains, bruises)	Use lowest effective dose for pain relief for shortest duration of time (known to increase risk of adverse GI side effects and may compromise existing renal function) Do not apply to wounds, eyes, or mucous membranes	Strongly recommended for knee OA Conditionally recommended for hand OA Insufficient data on hip OA Apply up to 4 times a day, fewer if patient is on anticoagulants or has chronic kidney disease

(continued on next page)

Table 1 (continued)			
Treatment	**Indications**	**Safety Considerations**	**Recent Guidelines**
Oral medications			
Acetaminophen	Minor pain and aches	Consider all sources, not to exceed 3 g/d Monitor liver function	Conditionally recommended for knee, hip, and hand OA Limited efficacy for cLBP and not recommended for routine use[36]
NSAIDs	Inflammatory diseases including tendinitis; mild to moderate osteoarthritis pain	Use lowest effective dose for pain relief for shortest duration of time Monitor for potential adverse GI, cardiovascular, and renal side effects	Beer criteria recommends avoiding chronic use of NSAIDs and completely avoiding use of indomethacin and ketorolac in older patients[37] Use should only be considered if there are no viable alternatives, and the patient can lower their risk of GI bleeding with use of a proton pump inhibitor or misoprostol[37]
Tramadol	Severe pain for which nonopioid analgesics are inadequate	Monitor sodium concentration (potential risk of SIADH or hyponatremia) and respiratory depression Complex effect on cytochrome P-450 3A4 inducers, 3A4 inhibitors, or 2D6 inhibitors	Beer criteria recommends to avoid extended release formulations and to reduce the dose of immediate release formulations[37] Conditionally recommended for knee, hip, and hand OA
Opioids	Acute or chronic moderate to severe pain for which nonopioid analgesics are inadequate	Use lowest effective dose for pain relief for shortest duration of time Monitor for respiratory depression (particularly in patients on benzodiazepines or gabapentinoid medications concurrently) Potential effect on cytochrome P-450 3A4 inducers or 3A4 inhibitors	Conditionally recommended against knee, hip, and OA, except when alternatives have been exhausted

Duloxetine	Neuropathic pain, central sensitization to pain, other persistent pain	Monitor serum sodium Risk of hyponatremia	Conditionally recommended for knee/hip/hand OA[35] Recommended for fibromyalgia[38] Consider for use in cLBP
Gabapentin/pregabalin	Neuropathic pain, central sensitization to pain	Can have sedating effects and cause dizziness Potential to have adverse effects on mood	Recommended for fibromyalgia[38]

Abbreviations: CNS, central nervous system; GI, gastrointestinal; NSAID, nonsteroidal anti-inflammatory drug; OA, osteoarthritis; SIADH, syndrome of inappropriate antidiuretic hormone.
From Refs.[35–38]

and prior trauma.[40] Although historically described as "wear and tear" of the joints, the pathophysiology of OA is appreciated as a complex interplay of inflammation, prior trauma, biochemical reactions, and metabolic derangements.[41] OA most commonly affects the knees, lower vertebrae, hand, and hips. Clinically, patients present with pain, impaired joint mobility, enlarging joints, swollen joints, crepitus, and locking or clicking of the joint.

The diagnosis of OA is usually based on history and examination. Identifying functional impairment should be part of routine assessment, and one should consider use of assistive devices and orthotics when appropriate to help preserve function and improve pain. Recent guidelines do not recommend laboratory data or routine radiographs to diagnose or monitor classic presentations of OA, although it is useful in atypical presentations.

Current evidenced-based guidelines of OA recommend a comprehensive approach that emphasizes nonpharmacologic therapies.[35] As highlighted in **Fig. 1**, exercise is also a core component of OA management. Exercise combined with dietary change yield a synergistic effect on improvement in pain and function, and it seems that the benefits in pain and function increase as the amount of weight loss increases in overweight and obese adults.[42] The specific exercises must be tailored to the individual's abilities and preferences, although a joint-preserving strategy should be used, with consideration for low-impact activities. Other nonpharmacologic options include behavior-based therapies (eg, cognitive behavioral therapy) and complementary, alternative, and mind-body approaches (eg, tai chi).

Pharmacologic treatment, listed in **Table 1**, includes offering topical therapies before oral therapies given the relative safety and side effect profile.[35] Topical nonsteroidal anti-inflammatory drugs do not carry the high risk for renal and gastrointestinal sequelae like their systemic counterparts.[43] Glucosamine and chondroitin products have limited utility for OA pain.[35] Intra-articular steroid injections are used safely on an as-needed basis, although frequent dosing regimens of every 3 months have not been shown to improve pain over placebo and are also associated with increased decline of knee cartilage volume on MRI.[44] There is mixed evidence of the efficacy of hyaluronic acid and hyaluronan polymer injections for the knee.[45] Whenever performing an injection, one should also inquire about concurrent use of anticoagulants and take measures to minimize bleeding risk.

Surgical arthroplasty of an affected joint is considered in select patients with OA-related functional impairments who have failed conservative therapies. Older adults experience a higher rate of postoperative complications compared with younger patients but have similar benefits in quality of life,[46] which highlights the need for evaluation on an individual level with shared decision-making between patient and physician.

Chronic Low Back Pain

cLBP is exceedingly common in older adults with prevalence estimates ranging between 10% and 20% in adults greater than or equal to 65 years old worldwide.[47] Most cLBP does not have one definitive cause. Rather, cLBP can be thought of as a common final phenotypic pathway that is a result of several possible contributors, including spinal stenosis, hip OA, sacroiliac joint pathology, leg-length discrepancy, myofascial pain, maladaptive coping, anxiety, and depression.[14] Assessment follows the domains listed in **Box 1** and must rule out infection, malignancy, and cord compression in a patient who presents with red-flag symptoms. The physical examination and imaging for cLBP should be used to investigate for sources of pain including the hips, sacroiliac joints, and vertebrae (see series on Deconstructing

Back Pain in Older Adults for distinct algorithms based on major presenting signs and symptoms).[48–50]

Successful management of cLBP involves various therapeutic modalities to optimize function, and begins with nonpharmacologic and rehabilitative modalities as depicted in **Fig. 1**. Physical therapy referrals should be recommended early and often. Referral to surgical specialties for spine is appropriate with any concern for central neurologic compromise or when neurologic deficits correlate with radiographic findings and/or conservative therapies have failed to provide significant improvement.

Crystal Arthritis: Gout and Pseudogout

Gout is a form of crystal arthritis characterized by an inflammatory reaction to monosodium urate in the joint. It is the most common inflammatory arthropathy in older adults and continues to increase in prevalence, likely caused by the relationship of hyperuricemia with hypertension, metabolic syndrome, renal insufficiency, and diuretic use.[51] Conventionally thought of as a disease affecting middle-aged men, elderly-onset gout (EOG) is also common and can present with unique features. Notably in EOG, women are affected at higher rates by gout older than the age of 80.[52] Unlike traditional gout, an initial gout flare in older adults more often presents with tophi, collections of uric acid in joints and skin. Conversely, podagra, painful swelling of the first metatarsal phalangeal joint, is less common in EOG. EOG is more likely to affect smaller joints of the hands and multiple joints at once, which can make differentiating gout from rheumatoid arthritis (RA) in older patients more difficult. When evaluating for gout, one should keep OA, RA, pseudogout, and infection in the differential diagnosis.

The diagnosis of presumed gout is often made clinically, based on the episodic nature of acute flares, although elevated inflammatory markers and serum uric acid are helpful. The diagnostic gold standard remains identification of negatively birefringent needle-like monosodium urate crystals on polarized light microscopy of synovial fluid from an affected joint. Plain film radiography can help support the diagnosis of gout, specifically erosive changes and overhanging edges of joints with preservation of joint space.

For gout flares, colchicine or corticosteroids are considered for treatment in the context of the risks to the patient and their comorbidities. Indomethacin should be avoided in older adults.[37] Intra-articular steroids are a viable treatment of flares involving a few joints and pose lower risk of side effects compared with systemic steroids. Longer-term preventative therapy includes lifestyle modifications and urate-lowering therapy in certain circumstances. Patients should be counseled to reduce or eliminate intake of alcohol, shellfish, and organ meats. Urate-lowering therapy is indicated for patients who suffer from more than two flares per year, have nephrocalcinosis, or present with tophi or erosions on imaging.[53] The goal uric acid level should be less than 6 mg/dL, and the initial choice of urate-lowering therapy should be allopurinol. In patients with chronic kidney disease, one can initiate allopurinol at the lowest dose and titrate to a target uric acid level while monitoring for adverse reactions.[54] Febuxostat, an alternative xanthine oxidase inhibitor, may be associated with increased cardiovascular adverse effects based on data from a single clinical trial.[55] When starting urate-lowering therapy, a patient should be on a prophylactic low dose of either corticosteroids or colchicine to prevent a "mobilization flare," which is when initiation of urate-lowering therapy can paradoxically trigger an acute gout attack. Gout can typically be managed by a patient's primary care physician, although one should consider referral to a rheumatologist if the patient continues to experience significant signs or symptoms of gout despite being on appropriate therapy, unclear source of hyperuricemia, difficulty in reaching goal serum uric acid level, or multiple and/or serious adverse effects from pharmacologic urate-lowering therapy.[53]

Similar to gout, calcium pyrophosphate deposition disease, or "pseudogout," is a form of crystal arthritis characterized by an inflammatory reaction to deposition of calcium pyrophosphate into cartilaginous structure of the joint. Pseudogout has prevalence rates of about 5% to 15% for adults older than 60 years old.[56] Age is a strong risk factor for pseudogout, and secondary causes include hypomagnesemia, hypercalcemia, hyperparathyroidism, and hemochromatosis. Acute pseudogout commonly presents as intermittent arthritis of the knee, wrist, or hand, although the axial skeleton can be affected. Like gout, the definitive diagnosis of pseudogout involves identification of crystals on synovial fluid microscopy; calcium pyrophosphate crystals appear as weakly positively birefringent rhomboid crystals in polarized light. Plain films are useful to aid in diagnosis when a patient is symptomatic, because chondrocalcinosis is often identified, although this can be an incidental finding in asymptomatic patients. Treatment of pseudogout flares similarly involves use of a course of steroids or colchicine. There is no medication specifically targeted to reduce the occurrence of calcium pyrophosphate deposition disease attacks but one should address reversible causes.

Rheumatoid Arthritis

RA is an autoimmune inflammatory arthritis characterized by progressive damage of synovial-lined joints and can include extra-articular manifestations. The prevalence of RA in adults greater than 60 years of age is about 2%, and incidence of RA peaks in the eighth decade of life.[57] Elderly-onset RA (EORA), defined as RA with onset after the age of 65, has several unique features, including equal gender distribution; greater incidence of larger joint involvement, such as the shoulders and hips; and lower rates of rheumatoid factor positivity. EORA may follow a more indolent clinical course, although this is not always the case. Patients usually present with multiple painful and swollen joints in a symmetric distribution.

Diagnosis of RA is based on history and physical examination with laboratory data and imaging used to confirm clinical suspicion. One should investigate for extra-articular manifestations, including rheumatoid nodules, vasculitis, and interstitial lung disease, as these portend a worse prognosis. Laboratory work-up should include rheumatoid factor, anti-cyclic citrullinated peptide (CCP) antibody, inflammatory markers, complete blood count, and complete metabolic panel. Joint arthrocentesis is not essential for diagnosis but is useful to help rule out crystal arthritis or infection. Classic radiographic findings of RA include decreased joint space width, juxta-articular osteopenia or osteoporosis, and erosions. There are no specific diagnostic criteria for EORA; however, the American College of Rheumatology (ACR) and the European League Against Rheumatism (EULAR) diagnostic criteria for RA are used.[58]

A cornerstone of treatment of RA is disease-modifying antirheumatic drugs (DMARDs), used in a treat-to-target approach, aiming to reduce the activity of disease and prevent deformity. Depending on severity of the presenting disease, patients are started on monotherapy or combination DMARD therapy, which often includes methotrexate, hydroxychloroquine, sulfasalazine, and leflunomide. Biologic therapies are often used after a trial of nonbiologic DMARDS and now include different targets (eg, tumor necrosis factor-α, interleukin-6, JAK, CD20).[59] DMARDS must be monitored closely for adverse effects including atypical infections and reactivation (tuberculosis or viral hepatitis). Corticosteroids are sometimes used at a low dose for a short period for active RA but should be avoided as a long-term treatment. Cardiovascular events are the leading cause of death in patients with RA, including older patients with

RA. A patient with suspected RA should be referred to a rheumatologist as soon as possible for early, aggressive management and monitoring of the disease.

Polymyalgia Rheumatica

Polymyalgia rheumatica (PMR) is an inflammatory illness classically associated with aching and morning stiffness of the shoulders, upper arms, hips, neck, and torso. It almost exclusively affects adults older than the age of 50 and has peak incidence in the eighth to ninth decade of life with a prevalence of approximately 1% to 2% for adults older than the age of 50.[60] Women are affected at about twice the rate than men. Patients can experience a symmetric polyarthritis of the hands, wrists, and knees, which makes differentiating PMR from RA challenging. PMR is a clinical diagnosis, and the ACR and EULAR have proposed classification criteria for PMR.[61] Because of its overlap with giant cell arteritis (GCA), every patient with PMR should be screened for GCA. Laboratory studies typically show elevated inflammatory markers with negative autoantibodies. Imaging is not required to make a diagnosis of PMR. The mainstay of treatment of PMR is low-dose systemic glucocorticoids. Physical therapy is useful to maintain function for patients with disabling stiffness and pain.

Giant Cell Arteritis

GCA is a vasculitis affecting large-vessel and cranial arteries with a peak age incidence in the 70s. Its prevalence is estimated at 0.7%, with similar higher rates in women like that of in PMR.[62] A reported 10% of patients with PMR develop GCA.[63] Common symptoms include jaw claudication, changes in vision, and dysphagia, and the feared consequence of untreated GCA is irreversible blindness. The gold standard for diagnosing GCA is a temporal artery biopsy of a section at least 1 cm long with multiple sites examined. MRI, PET/computed tomography, and ultrasound can reliably identify affected vessels but cannot definitively diagnose the disease. The mainstay of treatment is high-dose systemic steroids, which should be started empirically even before confirming the diagnosis with biopsy; diagnostic yield of biopsy remains high, even if the sample is collected after initiation of steroids. The Food and Drug Administration has recently approved the interleukin-6 biologic inhibitor tocilizumab for treatment of GCA, providing a steroid-sparing option. GCA requires expedient evaluation and management by a rheumatologist and often ophthalmologist. PMR can often be managed by the primary care provider unless there are more atypical circumstances, such as substandard response to steroids, unusual presentation, or difficulty tapering steroids.

Fibromyalgia

Fibromyalgia, also referred to as central pain syndrome, is a disease characterized by increased sensitivity to pain and often presents with fatigue, mental fogginess, and sleep disturbances among other symptoms. It is identified as a centralized pain state, where individuals have abnormalities in pain processing, although changes in peripheral pain processing also have been implicated. There is no singular cause of fibromyalgia; it is the result of a complex interplay of biopsychosocial factors. Estimates of prevalence in older adults is 2% to 4%, with women being affected two times as frequently as men.[64] The diagnosis of fibromyalgia is made clinically and follows the 2011 ACR diagnostic survey criteria, wherein a patient identifies widespread pain in addition to other symptoms including fatigue, depression, headache, and cramps.[38] Because of the widespread distribution of pain, the differential diagnosis of fibromyalgia is expansive and may be particularly challenging in older adults with multimorbidity. One must be careful to evaluate for other causes of pain, while understanding that fibromyalgia commonly coexists in the setting of other rheumatic diseases (systemic lupus erythematosus, OA, PMR, crystal arthritis, RA), myopathy, hypothyroidism, and vitamin D deficiency.

The recommended approach to treatment of fibromyalgia is similar to the approach depicted in **Fig. 1**. Although pharmacologic therapies may not improve function, they may improve pain, mood, and sleep. The class of medication demonstrating the greatest efficacy is antidepressants, and it is suspected that this is caused by the pain-modifying effect of increased norepinephrine and serotonin in central pain inhibitory pathways. Duloxetine and milnacipran, both serotonin-norepinephrine reuptake inhibitors, have Food and Drug Administration approval for pain relief associated with fibromyalgia. However, potential adverse effects include sedation, orthostatic hypotension, and urinary hesitancy. Pregabalin can also help improve pain symptoms and can be considered, although starting at a low dose given at nighttime and titrating slowly. Although tramadol and tricyclic antidepressants may help relieve symptoms, their use in older adults is not encouraged because of the adverse effects on cardiovascular and urinary systems.[37] Fibromyalgia is managed effectively by a primary care provider with a multidisciplinary, multimodal approach reflected in this review.[38] A rheumatologist may be referred if there is concern for inflammatory arthritis or underlying autoimmune disease.

SUMMARY

Persistent musculoskeletal pain in older adults is common, resulting in tremendous disability and cost to the individual and society. Later-life pain has its own unique challenges in assessment and management; however, it is a manageable condition with a multitargeted, multimodal, and multidisciplinary approach. There are still gaps in the literature to better understand and treat pain in older adults,[28,65] including broadening the evidence base for clinical trials for nonpharmacologic and pharmacologic treatments for musculoskeletal pain in older adults, because they are often excluded from these trials.[66] Another issue is access to evidence-based nonpharmacologic therapies. For example, cost and accessibility of physical activity programs or mind-body modalities have been identified as significant barriers to participation in an exercise program in older adults.[67] Taking the time to understand your older patient's pain experience (including diverse domains of sleep, social isolation, fatigue), by using a comprehensive assessment/evaluation, provides the underpinnings for an effective multimodal management plan and a strong, trusting therapeutic relationship. Listening to the patient and how they respond to therapies over time is the most valuable tool.

CLINICS CARE POINTS

- Obtaining a thorough history of a patient's level of pain, functionality, social engagement, and life at home from self-report or via proxy is central to evaluating possible contributors to pain and assessing resources available to aid the patient's therapy.
- Identifying referral processes and patterns with a diverse interdisciplinary team (as shown in **Fig. 1**) yields best results for complex older adults with musculoskeletal pain.
- Physical activity remains a cornerstone of persistent pain management. No specific exercise type has significant superiority over the other, which means that choice of exercise can be tailored to the patient's specific abilities and interests.

- A strong therapeutic relationship between patient and provider for effective pain management is defined by commitment by both parties, realistic goal setting, and availability of both parties.
- Using quantifiable metrics and goals, such as amount of time spent enjoying a (patient-identified) hobby per week, helps to gauge progress with pain-related therapies and can also help encourage the patient to engage and continue practicing therapies that are effective.

DISCLOSURE

Dr. Makris is supported by a VA HSR&D Career Development Award at the Dallas VA (IK2HX001916).

REFERENCES

1. Redfield RR, Kenzie WR Mac, Kent CK, et al. Prevalence of chronic pain and high-impact chronic pain among adults—United States, 2016. Morb Mortal Wkly Rep 2018;67(36):1–6. Available at: https://www.cdc.gov/nchs/nhis/index.htm.

2. Rundell SD, Patel KV, Krook MA, et al. Multi-site pain is associated with long-term patient-reported outcomes in older adults with persistent back pain. Pain Med 2019;20(10):1898–906.

3. Briggs AM, Cross MJ, Hoy DG, et al. Musculoskeletal health conditions represent a global threat to healthy aging: a report for the 2015 World Health Organization World Report on ageing and health. Gerontologist 2016;56:S243–55.

4. Lohman MC, Whiteman KL, Greenberg RL, et al. Incorporating persistent pain in phenotypic frailty measurement and prediction of adverse health outcomes. Eur J Pain 2017;72(2):216–22.

5. Blyth FM, Rochat S, Cumming RG, et al. Pain, frailty and comorbidity on older men: the CHAMP study. Pain 2008;140(1):229–35.

6. Chen Q, Hayman ÃLL, Shmerling ÃRH, et al. Characteristics of chronic pain associated with sleep difficulty in older adults: the maintenance of balance, independent living, intellect, and zest in the elderly (MOBILIZE) Boston study. J Am Geriatr Soc 2011;59(8):1385–92.

7. Karttunen N, Lihavainen K, Sipilä S, et al. Musculoskeletal pain and use of analgesics in relation to mobility limitation among community-dwelling persons aged 75 years and older. Eur J Pain 2012;16(1):140–9.

8. Whitlock EL, Diaz-Ramirez LG, Glymour MM, et al. Association between persistent pain and memory decline and dementia in a longitudinal cohort of elders. JAMA Intern Med 2017;177(8):1146–53.

9. Gaskin DJ, Richard P, Institute of Medicine (US) Committee on Advancing Pain Research, Care, and Education. Relieving pain in America: a blueprint for transforming prevention, care, education, and research. Washington, DC: National Academies Press; 2011.

10. Chodosh J. Quality indicators for pain management in vulnerable elders. Ann Intern Med 2001;135(8_Part_2):731.

11. Gibson SJ, Helme RD. Age-related differences in pain perception and report. Clin Geriatr Med 2001;17(3):433–56.

12. Blyth FM, Noguchi N. Chronic musculoskeletal pain and its impact on older people. Best Pract Res Clin Rheumatol 2017;31(2):160–8.

13. Murata S, Sawa R, Nakatsu N, et al. Association between chronic musculoskeletal pain and executive function in community-dwelling older adults. Eur J Pain 2017;21(10):1717–22.

14. Weiner DK. Deconstructing chronic low back pain in the older adult: shifting the paradigm from the spine to the person. Pain Med 2015;16(5):881–5.

15. Marengoni A, Angleman S, Melis R, et al. Aging with multimorbidity: a systematic review of the literature. Ageing Res Rev 2011;10(4):430–9.

16. Masnoon N, Shakib S, Kalisch-ellett L, et al. What is polypharmacy? A systematic review of definitions. BMC Geriatr 2017;17(1):230.

17. Zis P, Daskalaki A, Bountouni I, et al. Clinical Interventions in Aging Dovepress Depression and chronic pain in the elderly: links and management challenges. Clin Interv Aging 2017;12:12–709.

18. Blazer DG. Depression in late life: review and commentary. J Gerontol A Biol Sci Med Sci 2003;58(3):249–65. https://doi.org/10.1093/gerona/58.3.m249.

19. Chou KL. Reciprocal relationship between pain and depression in older adults: evidence from the English Longitudinal Study of Ageing. J Affect Disord 2007; 102(1–3):115–23.

20. Ickowicz E. Pharmacological management of persistent pain in older persons. J Am Geriatr Soc 2009;57(8):1331–46.

21. Guidance on the management of pain in older people. Age Ageing 2013; 42(suppl 1):i1–57.

22. Kaye AD, Baluch A, Scott JT. Pain management in the elderly population: a review. Ochsner J 2010;10(3):179–87.

23. Achterberg W, Lautenbacher S, Husebo B, et al. Pain in dementia. Pain Rep 2019;145(3):1.

24. Zwakhalen SM, Hamers JP, Abu-Saad HH, et al. Pain in elderly people with severe dementia: a systematic review of behavioural pain assessment tools. BMC Geriatr 2006;6(1):3.

25. Deyo RA, Dworkin SF, Amtmann D, et al. Report of the NIH Task Force on research standards for chronic low back pain. J Pain 2014;15(6):569–85.

26. Savva GM, Donoghue OA, Horgan F, et al. Using timed up-and-go to identify frail members of the older population. J Gerontol A Biol Sci Med Sci 2013;68(4): 441–6.

27. Jarvik JG, Gold LS, Comstock BA, et al. Association of early imaging for back pain with clinical outcomes in older adults. JAMA 2015;313(11):1143–53.

28. Reid MC, Eccleston C, Pillemer K. Management of chronic pain in older adults. BMJ 2015;350.

29. Makris UE, Abrams RC, Gurland B, et al. Management of persistent pain in the older patient: a clinical review. JAMA 2014;312(8):825–36.

30. Niknejad B, Bolier R, Henderson CR, et al. Association between psychological interventions and chronic pain outcomes in older adults: a systematic review and meta-analysis. JAMA Intern Med 2018;178(6):830–9.

31. Abdulla A, Bone M, Adams N, et al. Evidence-based clinical practice guidelines on management of pain in older people. Age Ageing 2013;42(2):151–3.

32. Taylor D. Physical activity is medicine for older adults. Postgrad Med J 2014; 90(1059):26–32.

33. Morone NE, Greco CM, Moore CG, et al. A mind-body program for older adults with chronic low back pain a randomized clinical trial. JAMA Intern Med 2016; 15213:329–37.

34. Hilton L, Hempel S, Ewing BA, et al. Mindfulness meditation for chronic pain: systematic review and meta-analysis. Ann Behav Med 2017;51(2):199–213.

35. Kolasinski SL, Neogi T, Hochberg MC, et al. 2019 American College of Rheumatology/Arthritis Foundation Guideline for the Management of Osteoarthritis of the Hand, Hip, and Knee. Arthritis Care Res (Hoboken) 2020;72(2):149–62.

36. Marcum ZA, Duncan NA, Makris UE. Pharmacotherapies in geriatric chronic pain management. Clin Geriatr Med 2016;32:705–24.

37. Investigation C. American Geriatrics Society 2019 Updated AGS Beers Criteria. J Am Geriatr Soc 2019;67(4):1–21.

38. Clauw DJ. Fibromyalgia: a clinical review. JAMA 2014;311(15):1547–55.

39. Barbour KE, Helmick CG, Boring M, et al. Vital signs: prevalence of doctor-diagnosed arthritis and arthritis-attributable activity limitation—United States, 2013-2015. Morb Mortal Wkly Rep 2017;66(9):246–53.

40. Zhang Y, Jordan JM. Epidemiology of osteoarthritis yuqing. Clin Geriatr Med 2011;26(3):355–69.

41. Mora JC, Przkora R, Cruz-Almeida Y. Knee osteoarthritis: pathophysiology and current treatment modalities. J Pain Res 2018;11:2189–96.

42. Messier SP, Resnik AE, Beavers DP, et al. Intentional weight loss in overweight and obese patients with knee osteoarthritis: is more better? Arthritis Care Res (Hoboken) 2018;70(11):1569–75.

43. Makris U. Adverse effects (AEs) of topical NSAIDs in older adults with osteoarthritis (OA): a systematic review of the literature. J Rheumatol 2010;37(6):1236–43.

44. Mcalindon TE, Lavalley MP, Harvey WF, et al. Effect of intra-articular triamcinolone vs saline on knee cartilage volume and pain in patients with knee osteoarthritis a randomized clinical trial. JAMA 2017;02111(19):1967–75.

45. Hunter DJ. Viscosupplementation for osteoarthritis of the knee. N Engl J Med 2015;372(11):1040–7.

46. Fang M, Noiseux N, Linson E, et al. The effect of advancing age on total joint replacement outcomes. Geriatr Orthop Surg Rehabil 2015;6(3):173–9.

47. Meucci RD, Fassa AG, Xavier Faria NM. Prevalence of chronic low back pain: systematic review. Rev Saude Publica 2015;49:1–10.

48. Weiner DK, Fang M, Gentili A, et al. Deconstructing chronic low back pain in the older adult—step by step evidence and expert-based recommendations for evaluation and treatment: part I: hip osteoarthritis. Pain Med 2015;16(5):886–97.

49. Lisi AJ, Breuer P, Gallagher RM, et al. Deconstructing chronic low back pain in the older adult-step by step evidence and expert-based recommendations for evaluation and treatment: part II: myofascial pain. Pain Med 2015;16(7):1282–9.

50. Fritz JM, Rundell SD, Dougherty P, et al. Deconstructing chronic low back pain in the older adult—step by step evidence and expert-based recommendations for evaluation and treatment. Part VI: lumbar spinal stenosis. Pain Med 2016;17(3):501–10.

51. Leonardis F De, Govoni M, Colina M, et al. Elderly-onset gout: a review. Rheumatol Int 2007;28(1):1–6.

52. Agudelo CA, Wise CM. Crystal-associated arthritis in the elderly. Rheum Dis Clin North Am 2000;26(3):527–46.

53. Khanna D, Fitzgerald JD, Khanna PP, et al. 2012 American College of Rheumatology Guidelines for Management of Gout Part I: systematic non-pharmacologic and pharmacologic therapeutic approaches to hyperuricemia. Arthritis Care Res (Hoboken) 2013;64(10):1431–46.

54. Stamp LK, Chapman PT, Barclay M, et al. The effect of kidney function on the urate lowering effect and safety of increasing allopurinol above doses based on

creatinine clearance: a post hoc analysis of a randomized controlled trial. Arthritis Res Ther 2017;19(1):1–9.

55. Cuenca JA, Balda J, Palacio A, et al. Febuxostat and cardiovascular events: a systematic review and meta-analysis. Int J Rheumatol 2019;2019:11–5.

56. Richette P, Bardin T, Doherty M. An update on the epidemiology of calcium pyrophosphate dihydrate crystal deposition disease. Rheumatology 2009;48(7): 711–5.

57. Crowson CS, Matteson EL, Myasoedova E, et al. The lifetime risk of adult-onset rheumatoid arthritis and other inflammatory autoimmune rheumatic diseases. Arthritis Rheum 2011;63(3):633–9.

58. Aletaha D, Neogi T, Silman AJ, et al. Rheumatoid arthritis classification criteria: an American College of Rheumatology/European League Against Rheumatism collaborative initiative. Arthritis Rheum 2010;62(9):2569–81.

59. Singh JA, Saag KG, Bridges SL, et al. 2015 American College of Rheumatology Guideline for the Treatment of Rheumatoid Arthritis. Arthritis Rheumatol 2016; 68(1):1–26.

60. Partington RJ, Muller S, Helliwell T, et al. Incidence, prevalence and treatment burden of polymyalgia rheumatica in the UK over two decades: a population-based study. Ann Rheum Dis 2018;77(12):1750–6.

61. Dasgupta B, Cimmino MA, Kremers HM, et al. Provisional classification criteria for polymyalgia rheumatica: a European League Against Rheumatism/American College of Rheumatology collaborative initiative. Arthritis Rheum 2012;64(4):943–54.

62. Crowson CS, Matteson EL. Contemporary prevalence estimates for giant cell arteritis and polymyalgia rheumatica, 2015. Semin Arthritis Rheum 2017;47(2): 253–6.

63. Narváez J, Estrada P, López-Vives L, et al. Prevalence of ischemic complications in patients with giant cell arteritis presenting with apparently isolated polymyalgia rheumatica. Semin Arthritis Rheum 2015;45(3):328–33.

64. Vincent A, Lahr BD, Wolfe F, et al. Prevalence of fibromyalgia: a population-based study in Olmsted County, Minnesota, utilizing the Rochester Epidemiology Project. Arthritis Care Res (Hoboken) 2013;65(5):786–92.

65. Makris UE, Misra D, Yung R. Gaps in aging research as it applies to rheumatologic clinical care. Clin Geriatr Med 2017;33(1):119–33.

66. Bowen E, Nayfe R, Milburn N, et al. Do decision aids benefit patients with chronic musculoskeletal pain? A systematic review. Pain Med 2020;21(5):951–69.

67. Bethancourt HJ, Rosenberg DE, Beatty T, et al. Barriers to and facilitators of physical activity program use among older adults. Clin Med Res 2014;12(1–2):10–20.

Osteoporosis in Older Adults

Catherine Bree Johnston, MD, MPH*, Meenakshi Dagar, MD

KEYWORDS

- Osteoporosis • Postmenopausal osteoporosis • Older adults

KEY POINTS

- Osteoporosis-related fractures of the hip, vertebra, and pelvis are a common cause of morbidity and mortality in older adults.
- All healthy adults should be counseled about measures to prevent osteoporosis, including adequate calcium and vitamin D intake, participating in weight-bearing exercise, and avoiding tobacco and excess alcohol consumption.
- Women should be screened for osteoporosis beginning at age 65. Screening for osteoporosis in men should be considered when risk factors are present. Appropriate screening intervals are controversial.
- Women and men with osteoporosis should be offered pharmacologic therapy. Choice of therapy should be based on safety, cost, convenience, and other patient-related factors. Bisphosphonates are often first-line therapy based on efficacy, safety, and cost.

DEFINITION

Osteoporosis is a disease characterized by low bone mass and disruption of bone architecture, resulting in compromised bone strength and increased fracture risk. Osteoporosis is also considered a silent disease, as there are commonly no symptoms until the first fracture occurs.

The World Health Organization defines osteoporosis using bone mineral density (BMD) and T score. T score represents a standard deviation (SD) that calculates how much a result varies from the average or mean bone mineral density of a healthy young adult. A T score of 0 means that BMD is equal to the norm for a healthy young adult. The more SDs below 0, indicated as negative numbers, the lower the BMD and higher the risk of fracture. Osteoporosis is defined as a T score of <−2.5. Osteopenia, or low bone density, is defined as a T score of −1.0 to −2.5 (**Table 1**).

Division of Geriatrics, General Internal Medicine, and Palliative Medicine, Department of Medicine, University of Arizona College of Medicine, Banner University Medical Center, 1501 North Campbell Avenue, Suite 7401, Tucson, AZ 85724-5801, USA
* Corresponding author.
E-mail address: Bree.johnston@bannerhealth.com

Med Clin N Am 104 (2020) 873–884
https://doi.org/10.1016/j.mcna.2020.06.004
0025-7125/20/© 2020 Elsevier Inc. All rights reserved.

Table 1 T score criteria for normal range, osteopenic range, and osteoporotic range	
Normal	Bone density is within 1 SD (T score +1 to −1) of the young adult mean
Osteopenia	Bone density is 1–2.5 SDs below the young adult mean (T score −1 to −2.5)
Osteoporosis	Bone density is 2.5 SDs or more below the young adult mean (T score <−2.5)

PREVALENCE

Worldwide variation in the incidence and prevalence of osteoporosis is difficult to determine because of problems with underdiagnosis. The best way to compare osteoporosis in different population groups is by looking at the fracture rates in older individuals. As osteoporosis is not a life-threatening condition, data from developing countries are scarce. Worldwide, osteoporosis causes more than 8.9 million fractures annually, resulting in an osteoporotic fracture every 3 seconds.[1] Osteoporosis is estimated to affect 200 million women worldwide:

Approximately one-tenth of women aged 60
One-fifth of women aged 70
Two-fifths of women aged 80
Two-thirds of women aged 90[2]

One in 3 women over age 50 years will experience osteoporotic fractures, as will 1 in 5 men aged over 50 years.[3]

Data from the 2005 to 2010 National Health and Nutrition Examination Survey (NHANES) suggested that in the United States, 16.2% of adults aged 65 and over had osteoporosis at the lumbar spine or femur neck. The age-adjusted prevalence of osteoporosis at either skeletal site was higher among women (24.8%) than men (5.6%). The unadjusted prevalence was higher among adults aged 80 and over (25.7%) than for adults aged 65 to 79 (12.8%). The age-adjusted prevalence of osteoporosis was highest among Mexican American adults (24.9%), followed by non-Hispanic white adults (15.7%), and was lowest among non-Hispanic black adults (10.3%). Asian ethnicity was not included in the data.[4]

NHANES also found that 48.3% of adults aged 65 and over had osteopenia or low bone density at the lumbar spine or femur neck. Women had a higher age-adjusted prevalence of low bone mass at either skeletal site (52.3%) than men (44.0%). Adults aged 80 years and over had a higher unadjusted prevalence of low bone mass (52.7%) than adults aged 65 to 79 years (46.7%). Non-Hispanic black adults had the lowest age-adjusted prevalence of low bone mass (36.7%), while non-Hispanic white and Mexican American adults had similar age-adjusted prevalence of low bone mass (49.4% and 47.3%, respectively).[4]

RISK FACTORS

Risk factor for osteoporosis can be characterized as potentially modifiable and non-modifiable and are listed in **Table 2**. Some common risk factors are discussed in more detail.

Diet

A healthy diet in childhood is an important contributor to peak bone mass, and maintaining a healthy diet can help reduce bone loss in later life. Adequate dietary protein, calcium, vitamin D, fruits, and vegetables have a positive influence on bone health,

Table 2 Osteoporosis risk factors	
Gender	Women are at higher risk than men
Age	Risk increases with age
Ethnicity	African Americans are at lower risk than Asians, Hispanics, and non-Hispanic whites
Family history	Osteoporosis in first-degree relatives increases risk
Body size	Small, thin-framed people are more at risk
Sex hormones	Amenorrhea Menopause and premature ovarian failure Hypogonadisim in men Thyrotoxicosis Panhypopituitarism Hyperprolactinemia
Body weight disorders	Body mass index <17 Anorexia nervosa Malabsorptive bariatric surgery
Calcium and vitamin D	A lifetime diet low in calcium and vitamin D is a risk factor for osteoporosis
Medications	Anticonvulsants Glucocorticoids (>5 mg/d of prednisone or equivalent for =>3 mo), GnRH antagonist/agonist, SSRIs, thiazolidinediones, aromatase inhibitors
Lifestyle	An inactive lifestyle or extended bed rest/immobilization
Cigarette smoking	Increased risk with consumption
Alcohol	Increased risk with excessive intake
Comorbid illness	Hypercalciuria Osteogenesis imperfecta Homocystinuria Hemochromatosis Glycogen storage disease Cystic fibrosis Celiac disease Cushing syndrome Inflammatory bowel disease Diabetes mellitus

while a high caloric diet has been associated with lower bone mass and higher rates of fracture.[5]

Alcohol Use and Smoking

A meta-analysis based on 18 prospective cohort studies revealed a nonlinear association between alcohol consumption and the risk of hip fracture. Light alcohol consumption (0.01–12.5 g/d) appears to be associated with a slightly reduced risk of fracture, whereas heavy alcohol consumption (>50 g/d) is associated with an increased hip fracture risk.[6]

Cigarette smoking is a risk factor for osteoporosis. Smoking causes reduction in circulating levels of 1,25-dihydroxyvitamin D and parathyroid hormone (PTH). Smokers have small but significant reductions in bone mineral density when compared with nonsmokers.[7]

Glucocorticoids

Glucocorticoid (GC)-induced osteoporosis is the most common secondary cause of osteoporosis. It is estimated that 3% of the population 50 years of age and older has used GCs, and this percentage increases to 5.2% in 80 years of age and older.[8] Thirty percent of patients with long-term GC use (>6 months) develop osteoporosis.[9] Bone loss is more pronounced in the trabecular bone, predominantly in the spine and ribs.[10] The increase in fracture risk is dose dependent, and the effect is at least partially reversible once the GC is discontinued.

Diabetes Mellitus

Type 1 diabetes mellitus is associated with low BMD, and the risk increases with the duration of disease. Data from Health Survey done in Norway showed a significant increase in hip fracture rates among females with type 1 diabetes (relative risk 6.9, confidence interval 2.2–21.6) compared with nondiabetic female patients. The mechanism of bone loss in unknown.[11]

Type 2 diabetes mellitus was earlier believed to cause increased BMD. These reports were primarily based on the concept of BMD and not from prospective controlled trials. Patients with generally larger body size and relatively high bone mass have higher fracture rates. Bone quality changes are related to microvascular events common in diabetes. A large prospective study of older women obtained from the Study of Osteoporotic Fractures, confirmed that female patients with type 2 diabetes experience higher fracture rates in regions of the hip, humerus, and foot compared with nondiabetic female patients.[12]

OSTEOPOROSIS COMPLICATIONS

Bone fractures are the most serious complication of osteoporosis. Fractures can occur at any bone site, but are most common in the hip and vertebrae. Fractures may lead to chronic pain, disability, depression, nursing home stay, reduced quality of life, and increased mortality. Pain from fracture is often the first presenting symptom of osteoporosis. Because of weakened architecture of vertebral bone, minor fractures over time can cause compression fracture. It can also lead to a condition called kyphosis, sometimes called dowager's hump. Vertebral fractures are the most prevalent osteoporotic fractures and are paradoxically the most underdiagnosed. Vertebral fractures are the predictors of future fracture risk; the probability is fivefold for subsequent vertebral fractures and twofold to threefold for fractures at other sites.[13]

Hip fractures occur usually after a fall. Hip fractures are associated with 15% to 20% increased mortality rate within 1 year, with a higher mortality rate in men than in women, followed by a 2.5-fold increased risk of future fractures. Approximately 20% to 50% hip fracture patients require long-term nursing home care and suffer from decreased quality of life, social isolation, depression, and loss of self-esteem.[13]

Multiple vertebral thoracic fractures may result in restrictive lung disease and worsened pulmonary function in women with pre-existing lung disease. Lumbar fractures may decrease the volumes between the ribs to the pelvis, alter abdominal anatomy, crowd internal organs (particularly the gastrointestinal [GI] system, causing GI complaints such as premature satiety, reduced appetite, abdominal pain, constipation, and distention); further, back pain (acute and chronic), prolonged disability, poor self-image, social isolation, depression, and positional restriction are other problems created by compression fractures in addition to increased mortality.[14]

NONPHARMACOLOGIC MEASURES FOR PREVENTION AND TREATMENT OF OSTEOPOROSIS

Once peak bone mass has been attained (ie, in middle and late middle age), the goal of prevention is to reduce the rate of bone loss. Prevention strategies include nutrition, exercise, and lifestyle factors.

Nutrition strategies include adequate calcium and vitamin D intake. The recommended calcium intake for postmenopausal women and men over age 70 is 1200 mg/d[15] Most adults do not require calcium supplementation. The US Preventive Services Task Force concluded that evidence was insufficient to recommend calcium supplementation for primary prevention (USPSTF).[16] The recommended intake of vitamin D is 600 to 800 IU daily, which can be difficult to achieve by diet alone.[17,18] Many older adults, particularly those with low dietary intake or those who are at risk of vitamin D deficiency (eg, homebound patients) benefit from supplementation. Screening for vitamin D deficiency is not recommended routinely in asymptomatic adults, but may be considered in patients at high risk for vitamin D deficiency. Although the ideal serum level of vitamin D is controversial, some experts recommend supplementation with a target serum level of 25-OH vitamin D above 20 to 30 ng/mL.[18]

Providers should recommend exercise to patients for multiple health benefits. Weight-bearing and/or resistance activity on most or all days of the week can help maintain muscle mass and BMD. Structured exercise and balance programs (eg, tai chi) can help reduce falls.[18,19]

All patients should be advised to eliminate or minimize the potentially reversible risk factors that have been discussed previously.

All older adults, but particularly older adults with osteoporosis, should be counseled in fall prevention strategies, including exercise, particularly strength and balance training, reduction or elimination of sedative-hypnotic medications, and environmental modifications.[15,18,19]

FRACTURE RISK ASSESSMENT TOOL

Risk assessment is most commonly conducted using the Fracture Risk Assessment Tool (FRAX), which is a tool that helps predict a patient's 10-year risk of hip or other major osteoporotic fracture. It has been validated for untreated patients aged 40 to 90 years in multiple countries and for multiple ethnicities. It can be accessed at www.sheffield.ac.uk/FRAX. Limitations of FRAX include that it is limited to only 4 ethnicities in the United States (Caucasian, Black, Hispanic, and Asian) and lack of validation in treated patients.[20,21]

SCREENING FOR OSTEOPOROSIS

The US Preventive Service Task Force and other societies recommend screening for osteoporosis in all women aged 65 and older.[15,18,19,22] Screening should be conducted at the hip and spine using dual energy-x-ray absorptiometry (DXA). Some guidelines recommend screening younger women with osteoporosis risk factors, but there is no consensus on how to optimally manage osteoporosis in this age group. Men should not be routinely screened for osteoporosis; however, they should be evaluated with DXA if they have risk factors for osteoporosis (eg, hypogonadism, androgen deprivation therapy, long-term glucocorticoid therapy, or celiac disease), loss of height, or fragility fractures.[15,18,19]

Screening intervals are controversial. One study suggested a screen interval of 10 to 15 years for older women with baseline T scores of >−1.5, 5 years for those with moderate osteopenia (T score < −1.5 and >>-2.0) and 1 year for those with advanced osteopenia (T score <−2.0 and >−2.5), but this is not a consensus recommendation.[23] When to stop screening is also controversial.[15] It is reasonable to discontinue screening if treatment would not be considered based on comorbidities or patient preferences, or if life expectancy is so short (ie, less than 1–2 years) that the patient would be unlikely to benefit from treatment.

DIAGNOSIS

The diagnosis of osteoporosis can be made in the presence of a fragility fracture, particularly at the spine, hip, wrist, humerus, rib, or pelvis without measurement of BMD can also be made in the presence of a T score of no more than 2.5 SDs at any site based on measurement by DXA. Several professional organizations also support making the diagnosis when the 10- year probability of a major osteoporotic fracture is greater than 20% or the 10 year probability of hip fracture is greater than 3%.[15,18,19]

Most experts recommend laboratory evaluation with a complete blood count, a chemistry panel that includes calcium, phosphorous, and alkaline phosphatase, and a 25-hydoxyvitamin D level. Further evaluation is indicated when there is suspicion for hyperthyroidism, celiac disease, multiple myeloma, hypogonadism, or hyperparathyroidism.[15,18,19]

TREATMENT

All men and women who meet the criteria for the diagnosis of osteoporosis should be counseled about nonpharmacologic preventive measures including exercise, diet, smoking cessation, and reduction of fall risk.[15,18,19]

Pharmacologic Treatment

Both women and men with osteoporosis should be offered pharmacologic treatment, although the evidence for benefit is stronger in women than in men. **Table 3** summarizes commonly used agents, dosing guidelines, adverse effects and precautions. Some guidelines recommend treating women with osteopenia with a 10-year probability of hip fracture of greater than or equal to 3% or a 10-year probability of any major osteoporosis related fracture of greater than or equal to 20%, while other guidelines suggest used a shared decision making framework in these situations based on patient preferences, risk profile, benefits, harms, and costs of medications. Reduction in fracture risk with pharmacologic therapy has only been demonstrated with diagnosis based on DXA in the osteoporotic range or with previous fragility fracture, not when a risk assessment tool such as FRAX is used.[15,18,19,24]

Evidence is insufficient to determine the comparative effectiveness of different pharmacologic agents for the treatment of osteoporosis; therefore, choice of therapy should be based on safety, cost, convenience, and other patient-related factors (see **Table 1**).[24]

The antiresorptive agents include bisphosphonates, denosumab, selective estrogen receptor modulators (SERMs), and estrogen/progestin therapy. Anabolic agents include the parathyroid hormone/parathyroid related protein analogs teriparatide and abaloparatide and the monoclonal antibody romosozumab.

Bisphosphonates

The bisphosphonates (risedronate, alendronate, ibandronate, and zoledronic acid) are effective therapies for established osteoporosis. To ensure optimal absorption, the

Table 3
Most commonly used osteoporosis drugs

	Efficacy of Fracture Reduction	Usual Dosing	Adverse Effects, Cost, Other Considerations
	Hip (H) Vertebral (V) Nonvertebral (NV)		
Bisphosphonates			As a class, osteonecrosis of jaw (rare) As a class, atypical fracture (rare, increased with longer duration of use)
Alendronate	H, V, NV	70 mg orally weekly	GI symptoms Generic is <$100/mo
Risedronate	H, V, NV	35 mg orally weekly 5 mg orally daily	GI symptoms $100–$200/mo
Zoledronic Acid	H, V, NV	5 mg intravenously yearly	Arthralgias, myalgias, headache, hypocalcemia, atrial fibrillation Generic <$100/mo
Ibandronate	V	150 mg orally monthly	Usually avoided because of lack of evidence of evidence for hip and nonvertebral fractures GI symptoms, cramps, myalgias $100–$200/mo
Other Antiresorptive Agents			
Denosumab	H, V, NV	60 mg subcutaneously every 6 months	Mild upper GI symptoms, rash, infections Increased risk of vertebral fractures after d/c Jaw osteonecrosis of jaw (rare) Atypical fracture (rare, increased with longer duration of use) $200–$300/mo

(continued on next page)

Table 3 (continued)			
	Efficacy of Fracture Reduction	Usual Dosing	Adverse Effects, Cost, Other Considerations
Raloxifine	V	60 mg orally daily	Thromboembolic events, hot flashes <$100/mo
Anabolic agents			
Teriparatide	V, NV	20 μg subcutaneously daily	Mild GI symptoms, hypercalcemia, renal events >$1000/mo
Romosozumab	V, NV	210 subcutaneously monthly	Potential for serious CV events Injection site reactions $1000–$2000/mo

oral forms should be taken in the morning with at least 8 ounces of water, in an upright position, with no other ingestions for at least 40 minutes. Even with these measures, there is a risk of esophagitis and upper GI symptoms. These agents are not recommend in patients with esophageal disorders or a creatinine clearance blow 35 mL/min 25-OH vitamin D, and calcium deficiency should be corrected prior to initiation of these agents.[15,18,19,24]

The intravenous (IV) bisphosphonates (zoledronic acid and abandronate) can be utilized for patients who cannot tolerate oral bisphosphonates (ie, inability to sit up for 40 minutes). IV bisphosphonates are sometimes associated with hypocalcemia and influenza-like symptoms.[15,18,19,24]

For patients taking bisphosphonates, most guidelines suggest reassessment of risk, including bone mineral densitometry, after 5 years of oral bisphosphonate therapy or 3 years of IV bisphosphonate therapy. Patients at continued high risk at 3 or 5 years because of low hip T score, a high fracture risk score, or history of fracture on therapy, should be considered for continued bisphosphonate therapy. The maximum duration of therapy is 10 years for oral bisphosphonates and 6 years for IV bisphosphonates. It should be noted that most data are based on osteoporosis in women, and data on optimal management in men are more limited.[15,18,19,24]

The risk of atypical subtrochanteric fracture increases with duration of therapy. In 1 study, the rate of atypical fracture was 1.78 per 100,000 in women taking the drug for less than 2 years (number needed to harm >50,000), increasing to 100 per 100,000 in women taking the drug for 8 years or more (number needed to harm 1000).[25] Both bisphosphonates and denosumab are associated with the rare complication of osteonecrosis of the jaw, which is most commonly seen in patients with severe dental disease.[15,18,19,24]

Denosumab
Denosunab is as a human monoclonal antibody that acts on the key bone resorption mediator RANKL, thus inhibiting osteoclast formation and survival. It has been shown to increase BMD and reduce the incidence of fracture in postmenopausal women. The risk of vertebral fracture appears to increase following discontinuation, making it less attractive as a first-line agent. Denosumab should be considered when there is a contraindication to bisphosphonate therapy (eg, reduced creatinine clearance). Like

bisphosphonates, denosumab is associated with the rare complication of osteonecrosis of the jaw. It also is associated with an increased risk of infection, mild upper GI symptoms, and rash. Because of the increased risk of fractures following discontinuation of therapy, continuing therapy or administration of another agent following discontinuation should be considered.[15,18,19,24,26]

Selective estrogen receptor modulators
Raloxifene inhibits bone resorption and reduced the risk of vertebral fracture, but there is no evidence that it reduces the risk of hip fracture, and for that reason, it is considered a second-line agent. It has potential benefits in reducing the risk of breast cancer, but that it offset by an increased risk of thromboembolic events and hot flashes. It should be considered when the risk of breast cancer is high and there are contraindications to other agents. It is unclear how long SERMs can be safely administered; many clinicians discontinue therapy at 8 years because of lack of safety data beyond that time frame.[15,18,19,24]

Tamoxifen is used for the prevention and treatment of breast cancer but should not be used as a primary agent for osteoporosis. However, women receiving tamoxifen probably receive benefits in BMD.[15,18,19,24]

Sex hormones
Sex hormone replacement may help prevent bone loss in men and women who have other indications for their use (eg, hypogonadism in men, hot flashes in women), but should not be used for established osteoporosis due to lack of efficacy.[15,18,19,24]

Parathyroid hormone/parathyroid hormone-related protein analogs
Teriparatide and abaloparatide are anabolic agents that stimulate bone formation and activate bone remodeling. They are not considered first-line agents for most patients because of cost. They should be considered in women or men with severe osteoporosis (T score of < or = −3.5 or T score < or = −2.5 with a fragility fracture), in patients who are unable to tolerate other therapies, or in patients who fail other therapies. Adverse effects include mild upper GI symptoms, hypercalcemia, and depression. They should not be used longer than 24 months because of a potential risk of osteosarcoma (observed in rats). Patients at high risk for fracture following discontinuation should be treated with an antiresorptive agent.[15,18,19,24]

Romosozumab
Romosozumab is a monoclonal antisclerostin antibody that has been shown to increase BMD and reduce vertebral and nonvertebral fractures. In has been associated with an increased risk of serious cardiovascular events.[27] It should be considered only for patients who fail other agents and are at low risk for adverse cardiovascular outcomes. Therapy is limited to 12 monthly doses. Patients at high risk for fracture following discontinuation should be treated with an antiresorptive agent.[27,28]

Other agents
Bazedoxifine is a SERM that is used in Europe and Japan for women with osteoporosis. It is also used in combination with estrogen for the prevention of osteoporosis. It is not used in the United States for treatment of osteoporosis.[29] Calcitonin is no longer used to treat osteoporosis. However, it may have analgesic properties that can be helpful in the setting of acute osteoporotic vertebral fractures.[30]

Special populations and considerations
There is evidence that bisphosphonates and teriparatide are effective for older patients as well as younger patients.[24] In general, the evidence is insufficient to draw

strong conclusions about the efficacy of pharmacologic treatment of osteoporosis in men.[24] There is some evidence that alendronate, risedronate, and teriparatide are effective in patients taking glucocorticoids.[31]

CLINICAL CARE POINTS

FRAX helps predict a patient's 10 year risk of hip or other major osteoporotic fracture, and can help guide treatment decisions. Fall prevention strategies can reduce the risk of fracture in patients with osteoporosis.

IV bisphosphonate use should be reassessed after 3 years of use; only patients with significant risk of future fracture should continue. Six years is the maximum duration of therapy for IV bisphosphonates.

Oral bisphosphonate use should be reassessed after 5 years of use; only patients with significant risk of future fracture should continue. Ten years is the maximum duration of therapy for oral bisphosphonates.

The risk of vertebral fracture appears to increase following discontinuation of denosumab. It should either be continued indefinitely or followed by administration of another agent.

The risk of atypical fractures of the femur increases with duration of use of bisphosphonates and denosumab. The complication is rare but potentially serious.

SUMMARY

Osteoporosis and its associated complications are common causes of morbidity and mortality in older adults. All healthy adults should be counselled about measures to prevent osteoporosis, including adequate calcium and vitamin D intake, participating in weight-bearing exercise, and avoiding tobacco and excess alcohol consumption.

Women should be screened for osteoporosis beginning at age 65. Screening for osteoporosis in men should be considered when risk factors are present. Appropriate screening intervals are controversial.

Women and men with osteoporosis should be offered pharmacologic therapy. Choice of therapy should be based on safety, cost, convenience, and other patient related factors. Duration of therapy depends on agent chosen and the patient's risk for future fractures.

DISCLOSURE

Neither author has anything to disclose.

REFERENCES

1. Johnell O, Kanis JA. An estimate of the worldwide prevalence and disability associated with osteoporotic fractures. Osteoporos Int 2006;17:1726.
2. Kanis JA. Assessment of osteoporosis at the primary health care level. WHO technical report, vol. 66. Sheffield, UK: University of Sheffield; 2007. Available at: https://www.sheffield.ac.uk/FRAX/pdfs/WHO_Technical_Report.pdf. Accessed January 30, 2020.
3. Kanis JA, Johnell O, Oden A, et al. Long-term risk of osteoporotic fracture in Malmo. Osteoporos Int 2000;11:669.
4. Looker AC, Frenk SM. Percentage of adults aged 65 and over with osteoporosis or low bone mass at the femur neck or lumbar spine: United States, 2005–2010. Atlanta, GA: Division of Health and Nutrition Examination Surveys; 2015. Available

at: https://www.cdc.gov/nchs/data/hestat/osteoporsis/osteoporosis2005_2010. pdf. Accessed January 30, 2020.

5. Levis S, Lagari VS. The role of diet in osteoporosis prevention and management. Curr Osteoporos Rep 2012;10:296–302.

6. Zhang X, Yu Z, Yu M, et al. Alcohol consumption and hip fracture risk. Osteoporos Int 2015;26:531–42.

7. Brot C, Jorgensen NR, Sorensen OH. The influence of smoking on vitamin D status and calcium metabolism. Eur J Clin Nutr 1999;53:920.

8. Kanis JA, Johansson H, Oden A, et al. A meta-analysis of prior corticosteroid use and fracture risk. J Bone Miner Res 2004;19:893–9.

9. Gudbjornsson B, Juliusson UI, Gudjonsson FV. Prevalence of long term steroid treatment and the frequency of decision making to prevent steroid induced osteoporosis in daily clinical practice. Gudbjornsson B, Juliusson UI, Gudjonsson FV 2002; 61:32-6. Ann Rheum Dis 2002;61:32–6.

10. van Staa TP, Leufkens HG, Cooper C. The epidemiology of corticosteroid-induced osteoporosis: a meta-analysis. Osteoporos Int 2002;13:777–87.

11. Chau DL, Edelman SV. Osteoporosis and diabetes. Clin Diabetes 2002;20:153–7.

12. Ensrud KE, Ewing SK, Taylor BC, et al, Study of Osteoporotic Fractures Research Group. Frailty and risk of falls, fracture, and mortality in older women: the study of osteoporotic fractures. J Gerontol A Biol Sci Med Sci 2007;62:744–51.

13. Melton LJ 3rd, Achenbach SJ, Atkinson EJ, et al. Long-term mortality following fractures at different skeletal sites: a population-based cohort study. Osteoporos Int 2013;24:1689–96.

14. Siminoski K, Warshawski RS, Jen H, et al. The accuracy of historical height loss for the detection of vertebral fractures in postmenopausal women. Osteoporos Int 2006;17:290–6.

15. Ensrud KE, Crandall CJ. Osteoporosis. Ann Intern Med 2017;167:ITC17–32 [Erratum appears in Ann Intern Med. 2017;167:528].

16. US Preventive Services Task Force, Grossman DC, Curry SJ, Owens DK, et al. Vitamin D, calcium, or combined supplementation for the primary prevention of fractures in community-dwelling adults: US preventive services task force recommendation statement. JAMA 2018;319:1592–9.

17. Ross C, Taylor ST, Yaktine AL, et al. Dietary reference intake for calcium and vitamin D. Washington, DC: Institute of Medicine. National Academies Press; 2011.

18. Cosman F, de Beur SJ, LeBoff MS, et al. Clinician's guide to prevention and treatment of osteoporosis. Osteoporos Int 2014;25:2359–81.

19. Black DM, Rosen CJ. Postmenopausal osteoporosis. N Engl J Med 2016;374: 254–62.

20. Centre for Metabolic Bone Diseases. FRAX WHO fracture risk assessment tool. Available at: www.shef.ac.uk/FRAX on 1/30/2020. Accessed May 1, 2020.

21. Marques A, Ferreira RJ, Santos E, et al. The Accuracy of osteoporotic fracture risk prediction tools: A systematic review and meta-analysis. Ann Rheum Dis 2015;74: 1958–67.

22. US Preventive Services Task Force. Screening for osteoporosis: U.S. Preventive Services Task Force recommendation statement. Ann Intern Med 2011;154: 356–64.

23. Gourlay ML, Fine JP, Preisser JS, et al. Study of Osteoporotic Fractures Research Group. Bone Density Testing Interval and transition to osteoporosis in older women. N Engl J Med 2012;366:225–33.

24. Qaseem A, Forciea MA, McLean RM. Denberg TD, for the Clinical Guidelines Committee of the American College of Physicians. Treatment of low bone density or osteoporosis to prevent fractures in men and women: a clinical practice guideline update from the American College of Physicians. Ann Intern Med 2017;166: 818–39.

25. Dell RM, Adams AL, Greene DF, et al. Incidence of atypical nontraumatic diaphyseal fractures of the femur. J Bone Miner Res 2012;27:2544–50.

26. Tsourdi E, Langdahl B, Cohen-Solal M, et al. Discontinuation of denosumab therapy for osteoporosis: a systematic review and position statement by ECTS. Bone 2017;105:11–7.

27. Lv F, Cai X, Yang W, et al. Denosumab or romosozumab therapy and risk of cardiovascular events in patients with primary osteoporosis: systematic review and meta- analysis. Bone 2020;130:115–21.

28. Bandeira L, Lewiecki, Bilezikian JP. Romosozumab for the treatment of osteoporosis. Expert Opin Biol Ther 2017;17:255–63.

29. Peng L, Luo Q, Lu H. Efficacy and safety of bazedoxifine in postmenopausal women with osteoporosis: a systematic review and meta-analysis. Medicine 2017;96:e8659–65.

30. Knopp-Sihota JA1, Newburn-Cook CV, Homik J, et al. Calcitonin for treating acute and chronic pain of recent and remote osteoporotic vertebral compression fractures: a systematic review and meta-analysis. Osteoporos Int 2012;23:17–38.

31. Adami G, Saag KG. Glucocorticoid-induced osteoporosis: 2019 concise clinical review. Osteoporos Int 2019;30:1145–56.

Evaluation and Management of Difficult Symptoms in Older Adults in Primary Care

Chitra Hamilton, MD, Colleen Christmas, MD*

KEYWORDS

- Leg cramps • Dizziness • Vertigo • Insomnia • Weight loss

KEY POINTS

- Nocturnal leg cramps are best treated with nonpharmacologic approaches.
- Dizziness can be further distinguished into categories of vertigo, disequilibrium, presyncope, and nonspecific dizziness to guide further evaluations.
- Sleep and cognitive function are clearly linked, but whether sleep interventions significantly improve cognition in age-related changes in sleep has not been shown.
- Evaluation of weight loss in the elderly focuses on finding and fixing those contributors that are readily identified and remedied.

INTRODUCTION

One of the most challenging, and rewarding, components of caring for older adults is the complex decision making involved in determining how much of a given concern is to be expected with aging of the human body alone and not amenable (or even harmful) to treatments versus a vague or nonspecific presentation of a disease that, once identified and treated, leads to important improvements in health and well-being. This article discusses 4 common vexing symptoms in primary care settings with guides for what further considerations may guide evaluation and potential treatments.

LEG CRAMPS
Background

Nocturnal leg cramps (NLCs) are a common but poorly understood problem that affects up to 50% of the population more than 50 years of age.[1] NLCs increase with age in both severity and frequency and have been associated with decreased quality

Division of Geriatric Medicine and Gerontology, Johns Hopkins School of Medicine, 4940 Eastern Avenue, MFL Center Tower 2nd Floor, Geriatrics Suite, Baltimore, MD 21224, USA
* Corresponding author.
E-mail address: cchristm@jhmi.edu
Twitter: @ChitraHamilton (C.H.); @CchristmColleen (C.C.)

Med Clin N Am 104 (2020) 885–894
https://doi.org/10.1016/j.mcna.2020.06.008
0025-7125/20/© 2020 Elsevier Inc. All rights reserved.

of life and reduced quality of sleep.[2] Often described as a musculoskeletal disorder, NLCs are characterized by episodic, persistently painful, involuntary muscle tightness, most often in the calf, thigh, or foot, lasting seconds to many minutes. At present, no clear cause or mechanism of NLC has been determined, although there is some consideration given to shortened muscle length as a risk factor in older adults who are less physically active.

Electromyography has shown cramp discharges during NLCs, with a variability in firing rates from 40 to 60 Hz.[3] The muscle discharges occur in a sputtering fashion with abrupt onset and cessation, distinguishing them from dystonia or voluntary muscle contraction.

NLC can be idiopathic or secondary to other causes, such as structural/mechanical causes, neurologic disorders, or metabolic/fluid disturbances. Structural or mechanical causes include genu recurvatum, flat feet, or prolonged sitting. Neurologic conditions such as Parkinson disease, multiple sclerosis, motor neuron disease, and nerve root compression can predispose patients to NLC. Metabolic and fluid/electrolyte causes include extracellular volume depletion, dialysis disequilibrium syndrome, hypoglycemia, hypomagnesemia, and hypocalcemia. Most commonly, patients have no evidence of volume depletion or electrolyte imbalances.

Medications, a common culprit of adverse effects in the geriatric population, can also contribute to NLC. The most common of these include long-acting beta-agonists, potassium-sparing diuretics, thiazidelike diuretics, and donepezil.

Diagnosis and Differential Diagnosis

NLCs are often misdiagnosed because of heterogeneity of symptoms. Most often, patients present to their primary care providers complaining of insomnia or sleep disturbance but not necessarily with symptoms of NLC. Almost all patients have cramps in the evening. NLC may be seasonal and can double in frequency from winter to summer. The reason for this is currently unknown.[4]

As with any medical ailment, a focused history and examination is pivotal in making the diagnosis of NLC. Laboratory testing and other studies are typically not indicated. The focused history should confirm the symptoms and identify any possible predisposing factors or medication causes. Inspection of legs, feet, and pulses should occur. Lastly, a neurologic examination should include assessment of strength, gait, deep tendon reflexes, sensation to light touch and pinprick, and assessment of tremor.

The diagnosis for NLC as described by the American Academy of Sleep Medicine must meet all of the following 3 criteria: a painful sensation in the leg or foot associated with sudden, involuntary muscle hardness or tightness indicating a strong muscle contraction; the muscle contractions must occur during the time in bed, although patient may be awake or asleep; and the pain can be relieved by forceful stretching of the affected muscles releasing the contraction.

Because nocturnal discomfort or cramping sensations in the legs are common symptoms of other conditions, NLCs are often mistaken for other disease processes, such as restless legs syndrome (RLS), dystonias, peripheral vascular disease, or periodic limb movements of sleep. In RLS, patients also experience symptoms at night and may have a cramping sensation. However, unlike NLC, RLS is characterized by more continuous discomfort and a need to move the affected limb. A distinguishing feature of RLS is that it does not involve sustained muscle contractions. In periodic limb movements of sleep, the movements are involuntary and jerking. They do occur at night but are not associated with muscle tightening or pain. A formal diagnosis of PLM can be made with polysomnography. With peripheral vascular disease, cramplike pain can occur in a pattern of claudication, which is relieved with rest of the limb, unlike in NLC. Patients often have other findings of arteriosclerotic vascular disease, such as decreased pulses on examination. In addition, dystonias in the feet can resemble NLC because they can cause cramping episodes; however, unlike NLC, patients experience agonist and antagonist muscle cocontraction. The difference can be determined by electrophysiology studies.

Approach to Management

Treatment of NLC can be extremely challenging. Initially, nonpharmacologic measures rather than pharmacotherapy should be used. Stretching exercises in the weight-bearing position of the posterior leg muscles before bed can be helpful. Deep tissue massage, improved footwear, loose (not tucked) bed covers, stationary bicycle use in sedentary patients for a few minutes before bed, avoidance of volume depletion, ice massage, or hot shower or warm bath can be tried. During an acute cramping episode, patients should forcefully stretch the affected muscle, which can often provide rapid relief. All fluid or electrolyte abnormalities should be assessed and treated.

Many pharmacologic treatments have been unsatisfactory in prevention or symptom management. For many years, quinine derivatives were used as a preventive method.[5] Quinine has been associated with serious side effects, including thrombocytopenia, chronic visual impairment, blindness, and death secondary to cardiac dysfunction. In 2006, the US Food and Drug Administration (FDA) advised against off-label use of quinine for leg cramps.[6]

In patients with inadequate responses to nonpharmacologic interventions, medications such as vitamin B complex, vitamin E, calcium channel blockers, magnesium, and gabapentin can be used. Diphenhydramine has been used in some studies but, given the side effects in the geriatric population, this medication should be avoided. Vitamin B complex can be given at a dosage of 30 mg 3 times a day. Vitamin E can be given as 800 international units before bed. Iron may also be helpful in patients with iron deficiency anemia. Magnesium supplements are often marketed for muscle cramp prophylaxis and have been beneficial in pregnancy-related cramps.[7] Most recently, in a double-blinded placebo-controlled clinical trial, it was shown that oral magnesium oxide was not superior to placebo for older adults experiencing NLC.[8] Calcium channel blockers such as diltiazem or verapamil can be used, but, given concern for hypotension and falls in the geriatric population, these should be used with careful monitoring. Lastly, gabapentin at doses of approximately 900 mg/d divided between dinner time and bedtime can be used as a last resort, with particular care in older patients given the risk of side effects. If the patient is resistant to pharmacotherapies, the use of tonic water rather than prescription quinine can be used if cramps persist and are disabling and severe. In addition, if pharmacotherapy continues to be ineffective, in patients who experience significant distress from NLC, a referral to a sleep specialist may be made to clarify the diagnosis and to see whether there is another underlying sleep disorder.

DIZZINESS
Background

Dizziness is a broad symptom described by up to 30% of geriatric patients in the clinic setting. It has been estimated that primary care physicians manage more than 50% of the patients who present with dizziness. It is a growing public health concern because it causes falls, which is the leading cause of hospital admission in older patients. Because dizziness is a broad and complex term, it is most often broken down into different types, including vertigo, disequilibrium, presyncope, and nonspecific dizziness. The sensation of dizziness can be associated with changes in the sensory, vestibular, visual, neurologic, or musculoskeletal system, all of which decline with age. Dizziness in the elderly should be considered a multifactorial geriatric syndrome involving many symptoms from a variety of causes, including neurologic, sensory, psychological, cardiovascular, and medication-related problems.[9]

The most frequent form of vestibular dysfunction in the elderly is benign paroxysmal positional vertigo (BPPV), followed by Meniere disease.

Diagnosis and Differential Diagnosis

Given the numerous causes of dizziness, this article breaks down the diagnosis by various types. Work-up, including a good history and physical, usually leads to an appropriate diagnosis; however, it has been found that the final cause of dizziness cannot be identified in up to 20% of patients. In general, laboratory tests and radiography are not beneficial in the work-up of patients with dizziness if no other neurologic abnormalities are found on examination.[10] Presbystasis refers to dizziness without an attributable cause.

Vertigo

Vertigo is often described as an interpretation of motion of the environment or self-motion. Commonly the words spinning, moving, or tilting are in patient descriptions. The description of spinning is often unreliable; however, lack of spinning can be used to exclude vestibular disease. All vertigo is made worse with movements of the head, which can help discern vertigo from other forms of dizziness. The presence of nystagmus is also suggestive of vertigo. Nystagmus may not be visible at all times and may be unmasked with a provocative maneuver such as Dix-Hallpike. It is important to remember that bilateral symmetric horizontal nystagmus for a few beats on lateral gaze is normal and that pathologic nystagmus is more prolonged and asymmetric. The elderly population has a higher incidence of central causes of vertigo, approaching 10%, most often caused by stroke. Although symptoms are important to help distinguish the cause, the duration of symptoms and aggravating factors can be more helpful in discerning the cause. With regard to duration, vertigo does not last more than a few weeks, because the nervous system eventually compensates for the dizziness. Determining the true meaning of constant dizziness is important for accurate diagnosis because many patients describe frequent episodic dizziness as constant. Prolonged dizziness is likely psychogenic and not vestibular. In addition, it can also be helpful to further divide patients with vertigo into acute prolonged episodes versus recurrent spontaneous attacks versus recurrent attacks with positional triggers. Most often, acute prolonged vertigo is associated with vestibular neuritis or stroke, whereas recurrent attacks can be associated with Meniere disease or migraine. When attacks are recurrent because of positional triggers, the diagnosis is likely benign BPPV.

BPPV peaks around the age of 60 years and is typically diagnosed by the presence of episodic vertigo provoked by changes in head position and findings of nystagmus during the positioning maneuver. BPPV is caused by calcium carbonate debris (otoconia) that is dislodged from the utricle for a variety of reasons, including inner ear disorder, infection, or head trauma.

Meniere disease is thought to be a disease of middle age; however, drop attacks from otolithic dysfunction are more frequent in older people compared with the general population.

Epidemiologic data for vestibular neuritis are scarce. It is thought that the peak age distribution is between the ages of 40 and 50 years. Vertigo lasting for hours with difficulty ambulating is likely vestibular neuritis.

Disequilibrium

Disequilibrium is the sense of imbalance that occurs with ambulation. It can result from a variety of causes, including peripheral neuropathy, vestibular disorders, visual impairment, musculoskeletal disorders, and cerebellar disorders. This sense of imbalance is often seen in patients with Parkinson disease. Most often, patients with this form of dizziness can be identified with observation of gait and full neurologic examination.

Presyncope

Some studies have shown that almost 70% of geriatric patients have presyncope type dizziness. Presyncope is often described by patients as feeling faint or a near-fainting episode. Typically, the symptoms are short lived, seconds to minutes, and can be accompanied by diaphoresis, nausea, visual blurring, or lightheadedness. Pallor is often seen by bystanders. Cardiac review of symptoms should be pursued in the setting of presyncope.

Nonspecific Dizziness

Nonspecific symptoms are often caused by psychiatric disorders, including major depression, anxiety disorder, somatization disorder, and alcohol dependence. Nonspecific dizziness can also be related to hyperventilation in stressful situations. Nonspecific dizziness can sometimes follow head trauma or whiplash injuries or be found in episodes of hypoglycemia. Patients should also be asked about nicotine, alcohol, and caffeine intake.[11] A medication review looking for side effect causes from antidepressant medications and anticholinergics is important. Some medications can also produce dizziness as a symptom of abrupt withdrawal. At times, if the cause is related to anxiety, reproducing symptoms with hyperventilation can often be reassuring and therapeutic.

Approach to Management

Given the causes of dizziness in older adults, multifactorial disease management should be customized to the individual. Variable approaches exist, including medical treatment, prosthetic devices, and vestibular rehabilitation. Vestibular rehabilitation includes habituation exercises to reduce pathologic responses to provoking stimuli. Vestibular rehabilitation can be effective in people with dizziness caused by vestibular dysfunction, cerebellar dysfunction, or Parkinson disease. In addition to rehabilitation, various prosthetic devices have been created to help with balance in the elderly. Vibrotactile feedback devices provide augmented feedback through vibration while improving postural balance during standing and ambulation. Currently, no medication exists to improve or inhibit the age-related deterioration of vestibular function. Although a common medication often used for patients with dizziness, meclizine should be avoided in geriatric patients if possible. Given its antihistamine properties and that it can act as a vestibular suppressant, it often causes sedation, delirium, and ataxia in the geriatric population.

INSOMNIA
Background

Concerns about poor sleep quality and quantity are common among older adults. Even though a third of people's lives is spent sleeping, clinicians are only recently beginning to understand the complex and important roles sleep plays in health. Increasingly, there is emerging evidence that, during sleep, people's brains are conducting processes to remove toxins that accumulate during the metabolic process of the daytime work and during certain stages of sleep in which learning is consolidated. Therefore, sleep disruption is thought to be linked to cognitive problems common with aging, although whether sleep changes cause poor cognition, are caused by poor cognition, or are simply an epiphenomenon is not yet understood.

Factors that control sleep tend to change with even healthy aging. For example, the drive to fall asleep weakens as people become older, even for healthy adults. Similarly, levels of melatonin production decline and relation to light and darkness also decreases with aging. In addition, there are environmental and behavioral factors that contribute to more time indoors and less exposure to bright light, often combined with reduced levels of physical activity, all of which can confound sleeping issues in older adults. In healthy adults the normal sleep pattern is that, after sleep onset, there is a cycle of non–rapid eye movement (REM) sleep that progresses through stages 1 through 4, ranging from lighter to deeper sleep stages, lasting 40 to 60 minutes. After the second cycle of non-REM sleep, REM sleep is introduced. In general, deep sleep stages predominate in the first third of the night and comprise about 15% to 25% of the total nocturnal sleep time of young adults. However, light sleep stages increase with aging and deep sleep stages 3 and 4 decrease with aging; REM sleep is largely unchanged but may be slightly decreased. Some older adults only get from 0% to 3% of their total sleep time in the deep sleep stages even without any known pathologic sleep disorder. In epidemiologic studies, the duration of sleep declines approximately 27 minutes for each increasing decade of life. Therefore, lighter stages and lesser quality of sleep are remarkably common with aging, even absent any disease process.[12,13]

Insomnia Diagnosis and Differential Diagnosis

Sleep concerns are common in primary care settings and approximately one-third of adults at some point request sleeping medications, but only 5% to 10% of those meet the criteria for insomnia. Insomnia is defined as difficulty falling asleep, staying asleep, or nonrestorative sleep that results in impaired daytime functioning and exists despite adequate opportunity to sleep. It must also be persistent longer than a month and occur more than 3 times per week with a preoccupation with sleeplessness.[14] To evaluate sleep concerns, a careful sleep history can help distinguish primary insomnia from other causes of sleep concerns. In particular, clinicians want to understand the timing of the insomnia; what the sleep behaviors are with regard to the sleep schedule and environment related to that; the daytime effects of this poor sleep; and any comorbid psychiatric, medical, or other conditions. In the differential diagnosis of insomnia are other sleep disorders that have specific treatments: sleep disordered breathing, periodic limb movements of sleep, and RLS, to name a few. Sleep disordered breathing is the occurrence of hypoxia and apnea episodes during sleep that lead to repeated arousals and hypoxemia. This condition is more common in men than in women and is associated with hypertension, cardiac disease, and pulmonary disease. Often patients report that their bed partners complain of loud snoring or choking or pauses in respiration while sleeping. Treatments for this include weight loss and use of dental or mechanical devices, surgery to reduce obstruction, and continuous positive airway pressure devices. Periodic limb movements of sleep is a disorder consisting of clusters of repeated leg jerking during sleep, diagnosed by a sleep study. The primary treatment of periodic limb movements of sleep is avoidance of alcohol, caffeine, and tricyclic antidepressant medications and treatment with dopaminergic agents. Periodic limb movements are similar to RLS; however, RLS consists of dyses-thesias in the legs with the sensation of creeping and crawling or pins and needles that is only relieved with movements of the legs. The sensations most commonly occur when the patient is in a restful state and are treated with iron (for patients who have iron deficiency) and dopaminergic agents. In addition, sometimes reports of poor sleep are simply related to unrealistic expectations of sleep as people age. Many people report concerns about their sleep when the pattern is compared with a younger age, but, when probed, do not have daytime somnolence or other ill effects of poor sleep. Reframing sleep expectations can be helpful in separating these conditions from true sleep disorders.

Approach to Management

In treating primary insomnia, clinicians first should consider sleep hygiene and then in-crease to more intensive therapies such as cognitive behavior therapy for insomnia, and then consider the risks and benefits of sleep medications in highly select patient populations for short durations.[15] In evaluating sleep hygiene, first it is necessary to understand whether the patient follows a regular sleep schedule, bedtime rituals, and how much time is spent in bed relative to the amount of time sleeping. Clinicians also need to understand the timing and quantity with regard to stimulants: their expo-sure to light; timing of exercise; use of stimulants, including caffeine, nicotine, alcohol, and allergy medications; use of cell phone and other blue light–emitting devices; and so forth. It is useful to evaluate the environment to ensure that the patient has a safe and comfortable sleep environment adjusted to the temperature level that is preferred for the individual and where noise and other factors that disrupt sleep are minimized.

Once sleep hygiene is maximized, if sleep is still inadequate, consider treatment with cognitive behavior therapy for insomnia (CBT-I). Therapists specifically trained in this technique, when available, can have dramatic and lasting impact on improving sleep quantity and quality, as has been well shown in multiple trials using various levels of interventions. Recently, commercial products deployed using digital applications have come to market and hold tremendous promise for helping patients who do not otherwise have access to a CBT-I–trained therapist. Tai chi, practiced 1.5 to 3 h/wk, significantly improves sleep quality among healthy older adults and those with chronic conditions.[16]

There is little evidence to suggest that medications to treat primary insomnia result in improved daytime functioning or large gains in sleep quantity, although often pa-tients report satisfaction with the use of sedative medications.[17] Although sedative hypnotic medications approved for sleep are only FDA approved for short durations, they are rarely used that way. In contrast, there is mounting evidence that sleeping medications increase the risks of falls, poor daytime cognitive performance, and over the long term may be associated with overall poorer cognition. Thus the risks of these medications in most instances outweigh any potential benefits, and their use in the older population is strongly discouraged.

WEIGHT LOSS
Background

Although articles discussing weight loss in the elderly often include titles suggesting that malnutrition is underdiagnosed and undertreated, there is no gold standard for its diagnosis and, in many instances, no effective treatment exists. The challenge for clinicians is to understand when weight loss is the marker of a disease that, once identified and treated, will result in clinical improvement and improved weight and when, despite extensive investigation, no reversible cause is found to understand the risks and benefits of nutritional interventions to try to improve clinical outcomes associated with malnutrition, namely death, functional decline, decubitus ulcer outcomes, infections, and quality of life.

Diagnosis and Differential Diagnosis

Weight loss is a straightforward diagnosis. Patients are often concerned about weight loss owing to changing appearance with aging, particularly loss of muscle mass. These concerns should be confirmed by measuring change in weight. Significant weight loss is arbitrarily standardly defined as a loss of 5% or more of the body weight in a month or a loss of 10% or more of body weight in 6 months, exclusive of reduced edema from the use of diuretics or other intentional changes in body composition.

Treatment

After confirming the weight loss, a structured approach can help identify treatable causes. Notably, some nutrition guides suggest measurement of albumin, prealbumin, transferrin, and other protein markers as guides to diagnosis and treatment. These markers track very closely with inflammation but are not useful to titrate nutritional interventions. Evaluation begins by reviewing any changes in appetite, dietary intake, medications, mood, and physical functioning.

A reasonable approach to treating confirmed weight loss often begins with discontinuing any medications that may be contributing to poor appetite, trouble swallowing, dry mouth, taste changes, or inattention. Clinically, evaluate for depression, thyroid disorder, chewing and swallowing problems, and need for assistance with obtaining food and feeding, and consider the risks and benefits of investigations looking for malignancies if identifying such an issue would result in important prognostic information or potential interventions. Interventions include minimizing medications, ensuring access to a palatable diet, adjusting the ambience during meal times to minimize disruptions, and considering compensatory techniques when swallowing problems are identified. Living alone, social isolation, and loneliness are all associated with malnutrition. As part of the environmental evaluation, these risk factors should be screened for.[18] These interventions ideally engage a multidisciplinary team including nurses, family members, medical assistants, and speech language practitioners. Before embarking on potentially more burdensome evaluations and interventions, consider carefully the likely benefit of those evaluations and interventions and ensure they are consistent with the patient's goals of care. In 1 study, involving a geriatrician in discussion of goals of care at the time of consideration of placement of a feeding tube resulted in a 50% reduction in the use of feeding tubes without any change in 6-month, 1-year, and 2-year mortality.[19]

In patients who lose weight owing to dementia, strong evidence mostly from cohort studies fails to show any improvement in survival with use of feeding tubes.[20,21] Some cohort studies suggest that mortality may be higher in patients with dementia with chewing and swallowing problems who are fed by tube than in patients who are fed by hand.[22] The addition of oral nutritional supplements to reduce pressure ulcers in malnourished individuals has shown conflicting outcomes.[23] The use of feeding tubes is associated with increased rates of Clostridium difficile, aspiration pneumonia and pneumonitis, and peristomal infections; there is no evidence they reduce the rate of any infections.[24] Overall, 13% to 40% of people who have feeding tubes placed have minor complications, 0.4% to 4.4% have major complications, and 30-day mortality after tube placement is 6.7% to 26%. In a classic study of 100 frail nursing home residents, provision of an exercise intervention substantially increased muscle strength and function compared with nutritional supplements alone or control; the addition of a nutritional supplement to exercise provided no statistically significant improvement compared with that gained by exercise alone.[25]

In patients with weight loss when a brief search for treatable causes is not fruitful and careful hand feeding does not seem to improve the situation, often families (and facilities) consider a feeding tube. This time is the ideal opportunity to discuss overall goals of care because mortality is significant and not changed by placement of tubes in most instances.

DISCLOSURE

The authors have nothing to disclose.

REFERENCES

1. Abdulla AJ, Jones PW, Pearce VR. Leg cramps in the elderly: prevalence, drug and disease associations. Int J Clin Pract 1999;53(7):494–6.
2. Hawke F, Chuter V, Burns J. Impact of nocturnal calf cramping on quality of sleep and health-related quality of life. Qual Life Res 2013;22:1281-1286.
3. Daube JS, Rubin DI. Clinical neurophysiology. 4th edition. New York: Oxford University Press; 2016.
4. Garrison SR, Dormuth CR, Morrow RL, et al. Seasonal effects on the occurrence of nocturnal leg cramps: a prospective cohort study. CMAJ 2015;187(4):248–53.
5. Tipton PW, Wszołek ZK. Restless legs syndrome and nocturnal leg cramps: a review and guide to diagnosis and treatment. Pol Arch Intern Med 2017;127(12): 865–72.
6. USFDA_2012. Available at: https://www.fda.gov/media/75097/download, Accessed July 8, 2020.
7. Dahle LO, Berg G, Hammar M, et al. The effect of oral magnesium substitution on pregnancy-induced leg cramps. Am J Obstet Gynecol 1995;173:175–80.
8. Roguin MN, Alperin M, Shturman E, et al. Effect of magnesium oxide supplementation on nocturnal leg cramps: a randomized clinical trial. JAMA Intern Med 2017;177:617–23.
9. Tinetti ME, Williams CS, Gill TM. Dizziness among older adults: a possible geriatric syndrome. Ann Intern Med 2000;132(5):337–44.
10. Swartz R, Longwel I P. Treatment of vertigo. Am Fam Physician 2005;71:1115–22.
11. Goebel JA. The ten-minute examination of the dizzy patient. Semin Neurol 2001; 21(4):391–8.
12. Duffy JF, Zitting K, Chinoy ED. Aging and circadian rhythms. Sleep Med Clin 2015;10:423–34.
13. VanCauter E, Leuproult R, Plat L. Age-related changes in slow wave sleep and REM sleep and relationship with growth hormone and cortisol levels in healthy men. JAMA 2000;284:861–8.
14. Bloom HG, Ahmed I, Alessia CA, et al. Evidence-based recommendations for the assessment and management of sleep disorders in older persons. J Am Geriatr Soc 2009;57:761–89.
15. Buysse DJ. Insomnia. JAMA 2013;309:710.
16. Raman G, Zhang Y, Wang C. Tai chi improves sleep quality in healthy older adults and patients with chronic conditions: a systematic review and meta-analysis. J Sleep Disord Ther 2013;2(6):1–6.
17. Glass J, Lanctôt KL, Herrmann N, et al. Sedative hypnotics in older people with insomnia: meta-analysis of risks and benefits. BMJ 2005;331:1169.

18. Besora-Moreno M, Llaurado E, Tarro L, et al. Social and economic factors and malnutrition or the risk of malnutrition in the elderly: A systematic review and meta-analysis of observational studies. Nutrients 2020:12(3):737.
19. Swaminath A, Longstreth GF, Runnman EM, et al. Effect of Physician education and patient counseling on inpatient nonsurgical percutaneous feeding tube placement rate, indications, and outcome. South Med J 2010;103:126–30.
20. Meier DE, Ahronheim JC, Morris J, et al. High short-term mortality in hospitalized patient with advanced dementia: lack of benefit of tube feeding. Arch Intern Med 2001;161:594–9.
21. Mitchell SL, Kiely DK, Lipsitz LA. The risk factors and impact on survival of feeding tube placement in nursing home residents with severe cognitive impairment. Arch Intern Med 1997;157:327–32.
22. Mitchell SL, Kiely DK, Lipsitz LA. Does artificial enteral nutrition prolong the survival of institutionalized elders with chewing and swallowing problems? J Gerontol Med Sci 1998;53A:M207–13.
23. Reddy M, Gill SS, Rochon PA. Preventing pressure ulcers: a systematic review. JAMA 2006;296(8):974–84.
24. Bliss DZ, Johnson S, Savik K, et al. Acquisition of clostridium difficile and clostridium difficile-associated diarrhea in hospitalized patients receiving tube feeding. Ann Intern Med 1998;129:1012–9.
25. Fiatarone MA, O'Neill EF, Ryan ND, et al. Exercise training and nutritional supplementation for physical frailty in very elderly people. N Engl J Med 1994;33:1769–75.

Perioperative Care Strategy for Older Adults

Teresa S. Jones, MD[a],*, John T. Moore, MD[b], Thomas N. Robinson, MD[c]

KEYWORDS

- Geriatric • Frailty • Delirium • Advance directive

KEY POINTS

- Geriatric surgical care is an evolving domain of specialized care.
- Geriatric patients require a standardized preoperative, intraoperative, and postoperative approach to achieve improved outcomes.
- Development of a multidisciplinary team to oversee the care and provide support to the providers is a necessary component of the care model.

INTRODUCTION

Surgical care of older adults is rapidly developing as an integral segment of surgical care across all surgical specialties. Americans aged 65 years and older are the fastest growing segment of the population, and this group uses a disproportionate amount of the overall health care resources. Almost 40% of all inpatient procedures are performed on patients more than 65 years of age.[1] Older patients bring a complexity in physiologic, sociologic, and psychological issues that are challenging the current care models. To answer this challenge, groups, including the American Geriatrics Society and the American College of Surgeons, have developed guidelines for perioperative management of geriatric patients. This article defines this high-risk group for surgical providers and guide them through an evidence-based, efficient preoperative, intraoperative, and postoperative care encounter.

PREOPERATIVE CARE: ESTABLISHING GOALS OF CARE

Traditional initial evaluation of surgical patients revolves around identification of the surgical problem and the surgical strategy to solve the problem. Discussions center

[a] Rocky Mountain Regional Veterans Affairs Medical Center, Geriatric Research Education and Clinical Center (GRECC), VA Eastern Colorado Health Care System, University of Colorado School of Medicine, 1700 North Wheeling Street, Aurora, CO 80045; [b] Department of Surgery, Rocky Mountain Regional Medical Center Veterans Administration Healthcare, University of Colorado School of Medicine, 1700 North Wheeling Street, Aurora, CO 80045, USA; [c] Rocky Mountain Regional Medical Center Veterans Affairs Medical Center, University of Colorado School of Medicine, 1700 North Wheeling Street, Aurora, CO 80045, USA
* Corresponding author.
E-mail address: Teresa.Jones@cuanschutz.edu

Med Clin N Am 104 (2020) 895–908
https://doi.org/10.1016/j.mcna.2020.06.010
0025-7125/20/Published by Elsevier Inc.

medical.theclinics.com

on the technical aspects of the procedure, discussing recognized morbidity and mortality statistics and a decision about proceeding with the procedure. Personalized risk assessment based on multiple organ systems and physiologic parameters, diagnostic evaluations of critical physiologic systems to achieve optimization for identified deficits, and completing an informed consent are the usual elements of this consultation. This disease-centric, or organ-centric, evaluation process does not account for the patients' own values or wishes for their health and well-being. Defining treatment goals based strictly on disease-related and organ-related outcomes is suboptimal.

Establishing patient-centered treatment goals in surgical therapy revolves around the extension of the patient's healthspan or the quality of that healthspan.[2] Healthspan is defined as the length of time during which an individual retains health and well-being (often maintenance of independence of function or the ability to live independently are used as surrogates to represent health).[3] The concept of healthspan is in contrast with the idea of lifespan (**Fig. 1**). Lifespan is the chronologic time for which the patient is alive and does not take into account quality of life. Major operations can extend lifespan at the expense of decreased healthspan. This approach begs the question during the preoperative consultation for a major operation: "But at what cost?" For older patients, surgical morbidity and mortality are higher than in the general population because of a multifactorial combination of chronic disease and functional decline.[4] The intensity of surgical care in this group is high, with up to one-third of elderly patients undergoing surgery during the last 12 months of their lives.[5]

A key assessment in the initial preoperative evaluation for geriatric patients is a clear elucidation of their overall health care goals. These goals are best clarified if they are specific and personal, preferably expressed in the patient's own words. "I want to attend my grandson's high school graduation" or similar sentiments are best gathered through open-ended questions, such as "What can you tell me about yourself that will help me to take care of you?" The surgeon through this assessment, in addition to other aspects of risk stratification, can help inform patients and their families of the anticipated impact of the surgical procedure on symptoms, functional status, living situation, burden of care, and survival. This strategy helps the surgical care provider align operative treatment goals with the individual's overall health care goals.

It is important to reemphasize the need to align older adults' most valued virtues and desires with the anticipated surgical outcomes based on the accurate geriatric risk assessment. An establishment of healthspan versus lifespan concept is intrinsic to this discussion. Included in the discussion should be a realistic outline of long-term

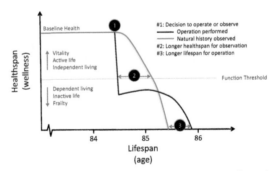

Fig. 1. Conceptualizing healthspan versus lifespan in the context of a major operation in the oldest old.

symptoms or functional limitations associated with the intervention; the time frames associated with the return to functionality; and the alteration in living situation, even temporary, that is either probable or possible. Most seriously ill patients (75%) say they would not choose life-sustaining treatment if they knew the outcome would be survival with long-term cognitive or functional impairment.[6]

Advance directives need to be obtained before major operative interventions in older adults. At minimum, a medical durable power of attorney's name and contact information should be documented before any planned inpatient operation. This information provides the clinical team with persons to contact postoperatively when patients do not have the capacity to make health care decisions for themselves. The named durable medical power of attorney should actively engage with the patient to understand what the patient's wishes are for life-sustaining treatments during a situation in which the patient does not have decision-making capacity. For more extensive elective surgical procedures with planned postoperative intensive care unit admission, the older adult's treatment preferences for specific life-sustaining interventions need to be documented in an advance directive document. Preferences for life-sustaining measures such as cardiopulmonary resuscitation with chest compression, intubation, feeding tube placement, blood transfusion, and hemodialysis should all be discussed, and the patient's wishes documented.[7]

PREOPERATIVE CARE: RISK ASSESSMENT

Historically, establishing surgical risk has relied on assessing and summing the presence of comorbidity, or chronic disease. The greater number of comorbidities present was subsequently equated to higher surgical risk. Ischemic heart disease is the most dominant comorbidity associated with poor surgical outcomes and therefore cardiac evaluation was the central focus of preoperative evaluation.[8] However, more recently, physiologic vulnerability in older adults has been recognized to be distinct from vulnerability in younger adults. The syndrome of frailty represents a distinct vulnerability in older adults that requires preoperative assessment.

Frailty better stratifies risk in older patients in contrast with simply summing comorbidity. Frailty is quantified by assessing a spectrum of characteristics unique to older adults.[9] The goal of a frailty assessment is to identify physiologic decline in older patients that forecasts poor surgical outcomes. A frailty assessment can provide management opportunities with the goal of improving surgical outcomes by directing preoperative and postoperative interventions directly at deficits discovered during the frailty evaluation (**Fig. 2**).

Age in itself is a factor that increases the vulnerability of the surgical population. The American College of Surgeons currently recommends using 75 years as the cutoff for high risk, because several studies have shown increased morbidity and mortality independently associated with age equal to or greater chronologic age.[10] Patients greater than 75 years old should be evaluated for additional risk related to frailty, including cognitive decline, impaired functional status, impaired mobility, and malnutrition.

Cognitive decline is evident in up to 24% of patients 80 years of age and older.[11] It is directly associated with multiple postoperative complications, including multiorgan failure and delirium.[12] Preoperative cognitive impairment can be quickly assessed by several screening tools, including the Mini-Cog test.[13] It is recommended that this assessment be performed and documented on all high-risk individuals to identify the abnormalities and to identify a baseline for comparison in the immediate postoperative period and for long-term evaluation.[7] Those patients who are identified with

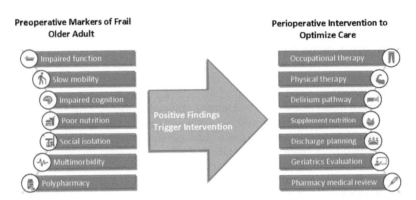

Fig. 2. Translating frailty evaluation into perioperative interventions to optimize care.

impairment should be included in a high-risk group and should have a delirium prevention bundle order set launched immediately postoperatively.

Functional status interruption is an expected occurrence before any major surgical procedure. Function is quantified by assessing the 6 activities of daily living: bathing, grooming, transferring, toileting, feeding, and continence.[2] Function is subsequently documented as independent if the patient is able to perform all 6 activities of daily living, partially dependent if the patient requires assistance in 1 to 5 of the activities of daily living, and completely dependent if the patient requires assistance in all 6 activities of daily living. Dependence in 1 or more activity of daily living is closely associated with poor surgical outcomes, including an increase in major complications, need for institutionalization, and mortality. The expectation of returning to the preoperative level of function may be unrealistic for some patients, a fact that needs to be discussed during the preoperative decision-making consultation. Although the most common tool to assess function is quantifying activities of daily living, assessment of instrumental activities of daily living (eg, ability to prepare meals, shop for food, and manage personal finances) is also a reasonable strategy for documenting function. The aspect of a true functional decline where the older adult never returns to the same level of function as the baseline exists. The trajectory of functional recovery for older adults is protracted compared with younger, healthy individuals and a return to baseline may never be achieved.

Impaired mobility is also a characteristic of frail older adults. Frail older adults' walking speed (termed gait speed) is slower than that of nonfrail adults. Multiple measurement tools exist to quantify impaired mobility. For surgical patients, the Timed Up and Go evaluation is an established and widely used strategy.[14] To measure a Timed Up and Go, the patient is timed rising from a chair, walking 3 m (10 feet), turning around, walking back to the chair, and then sitting in the chair. A time of 15 seconds or greater is closely associated with increased major surgical complications and greater 1-year mortality. Measurement strategies used as surrogates for walking speed in the surgical literature are the presence of 1 or more falls in the 6 months before the operation and the need for use of a mobility aid preoperatively.[15,16] Improvement in preoperative physical activity is associated with high likelihood to recover baseline walking capacity.[17] Multimodal preoperative strategies, termed prehabilitation, have been developed to initiate walking programs and nutrition assessment before surgery, and have shown decrease postoperative complications and reduced hospital costs.[18]

Nutrition assessment is critical because malnutrition is a common and under-recognized condition in the older adult population. Anorexia associated with weight loss and shrinking is a core characteristic of frail older adults. The reasons for poor nutrition can be related to factors beyond frailty-related anorexia; impaired ability to swallow and poor dentition are both recognized contributors to under nutrition in older adults. Nutritional status is important to surgical outcomes, because markers of pre-operative malnutrition are associated with increased postoperative morbidity.[19] However, up to two-thirds of older patients are at nutritional risk or malnourished at baseline, therefore initiation of nutrition in the postoperative setting should be as expe-ditious as possible.[20] For surgeons to recognize affected patients, it is recommended that a simple screening scheme looking for a body mass index less than 19 kg/m^2, weight loss greater than 10% to 15% in the previous 6 months, and a serum albumin level less than 3.4 g/dL as triggers for suspecting malnutrition.[7] Any 1 of these factors eliciting a positive response should generate a nutritional evaluation with institution of a preoperative and postoperative nutritional support.

It is important to reemphasize that the presence of 1 or more characteristics of frailty (impaired cognition, partially dependent or dependent function, poor mobility, and malnutrition) does not preclude an operation. These characteristics forecast poor sur-gical outcomes and that fact needs to be accounted for in surgical decision making. Early identification of the presence of frailty deficits aids in recognizing the need for early discharge planning. In addition, mitigation through management strategies designed to reverse the clinical deficit (eg, prehabilitation for functional impairment or nutritional supplementation for malnutrition) may be prescribed, although recent randomized controlled trials did not show a significant health benefit from aggressive intervention.[21]

PREOPERATIVE CARE: MULTIDISCIPLINARY TEAM DECISION MAKING

To aid in preoperative decision making for older adults considering a major operation, pre-sentation of all patient 75 years of age and older planning to undergo an inpatient elective operation is recommended. Establishing a multidisciplinary team allows the diverse input of specialists in the final decision to perform an operation. This strategy represents a sig-nificant departure from the traditional surgical decision-making pathway, in which an in-dividual surgeon decides with the patient whether or not to proceed with an operation. This care team is analogous to other such boards that are commonly found in most insti-tutions, such as tumor boards or preoperative transplantation committees.

The multidisciplinary team meets on a regular schedule to evaluate preoperative and postoperative care of patients 75 years of age and older with the goal of imple-menting evidence-based best practices for the perioperative care of geriatric patients. The membership of the multidisciplinary geriatric surgical team varies from institution to institution but generally includes geriatric surgical leadership, primary surgical team, palliative care, geriatrics, anesthesia, hospital medicine, critical care, nutrition, pharmacy, and social work (**Fig. 3**).[7] Documentation of the recommendations should be placed in the patient chart with communication to caregivers and families.[22] Before presentation of an older adult preparing for surgery at the multidisciplinary meeting, baseline assessment of frailty, patient goals of care, and comorbidity need to be docu-mented and available for the team to review. The primary surgical team commonly present their own patients being considered for a major operation.

PREOPERATIVE CARE: GERIATRIC-SPECIFIC SURGICAL RISK CALCULATORS

Surgical risk calculators are common tools used for preoperative decision making for any patient undergoing a high-risk operation. The most common risk calculator in use is the

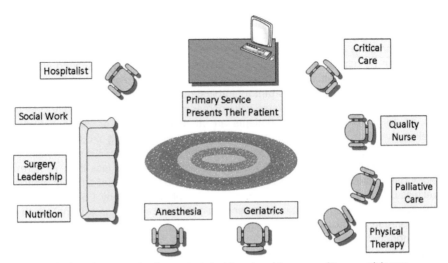

Fig. 3. Multidisciplinary geriatric surgical decisional-making committee participants.

American College of Surgeons risk calculator.[23] This tool is Web based, free, and easily accessible for clinical use. Preoperative baseline patient characteristics (eg, age, presence of specific chronic disease, function) and the proposed surgical procedure are uploaded into the calculator. In addition to the discrete input categories, providers can select a status button for low or high risk based on their own assessment, which may not be captured by the discrete input variables present on the calculator input page. After input of the preoperative variables, the risk calculator outputs forecasted outcomes for the individual patient compared with the accepted national averages for postoperative outcomes. Outcomes reported by the calculator include risk of 1 or more major postoperative complication, pneumonia, cardiac event, infection, and 30-day death.

Recently, the American College of Surgeons added geriatric-specific baseline variables and outcome variables to their widely used surgical risk calculator. Six additional baseline variables need to be input for risk adjustment: use of mobility aid, origin status from home, history of fall, impaired cognition, hospice care on admission, and competency to sign consent. The benefit of providing this additional baseline information is the subsequent outcome variables of postoperative delirium, decline in function, new use of a mobility aid, and progression of a pressure ulcer. This surgical calculator represents the first widely disseminated surgical risk assessment tool that accounts for the characteristics of the frail older adults and subsequently provides outcomes specifically relevant to the frail older adults.

INTRAOPERATIVE CARE OF OLDER ADULTS

The recommended intraoperative care of older adults does not significantly differ from the care of other adults. Specific management strategies important for older adults include:

1. Extra care in padding during patient positioning to prevent skin breakdown and nerve atrophy. Older patients are particularly susceptible to these injuries because of decreased skin integrity.[24]
2. Use of preemptive nonnarcotic multimodel preventive pain management strategies (eg, regional blocks, acetaminophen, gabapentin) before the incision to decrease anesthesia medications during the operation. General anesthesia in orthopedic

patients is associated with increased postoperative complications, including in-hospital mortality, length of stay, and readmission; however, the evidence is equivocal as to whether regional anesthesia is associated with improved outcomes.[25,26]

3. Avoid prescribing high-risk medications in the immediate preoperative phase of care (eg, routine use of high-risk antinausea medications) and intraoperative phase of care. For a list of commonly prescribed high-risk medications in the perioperative setting, see **Table 1**.

POSTOPERATIVE INPATIENT CARE OF OLDER ADULTS
Multidisciplinary Inpatient Care Team

The foundation of high-quality postoperative inpatient care of older adults depends on multidisciplinary team daily rounds focused on geriatric specialty care issues. Although the surgical and medical teams caring for elderly patients focus their efforts on the primary disease process leading to the current hospitalization, a multidisciplinary geriatric team is able to focus their efforts on issues central to optimal recovery of the older adults: functional preservation, delirium prevention, nutritional support, and discharge transition planning. The benefits of multidisciplinary team rounding for geriatric patients have been shown in multiple subspecialties, particularly orthopedic surgery, where there has been significant decrease in morbidity after surgery for geriatric patients as well as 30-day mortality and readmission rate.[27,28] Clinical pathways have now been developed that activate geriatric protocols beginning in the emergency department at the time of admission.

Table 1
Common perioperative medications with high risk of adverse events in older adults

Pain Medications	
Meperidine (Demerol)	Related to postoperative delirium
Indomethacin (Indocin)	NSAID with most CNS side effects
Pentazocine (Talwin)	Associated with hallucinations and confusion
Ketorolac (Toradol)	Increased risk of GI bleeding and peptic ulcer disease
GI Stress Ulcer Prophylaxis	
Cimetidine (Tagamet)	Anticholinergic properties predispose to delirium
Famotidine (Pepcid)	Anticholinergic properties predispose to delirium
Ranitidine (Zantac)	Anticholinergic properties predispose to delirium
Nausea Medications	
Scopolamine	Anticholinergic properties predispose to delirium
Promethazine (Phenergan)	Anticholinergic properties predispose to delirium
Insomnia Medications	
Benzodiazepines	Central nervous system toxicity, increase fall risk and fractures
Zolpidem (Ambien)	Increase risk of delirium and falls
Other Medications	
Diphenhydramine (Benadryl)	Anticholinergic properties predispose to delirium
Cyclobenzaprine (Flexeril)	Drowsiness, confusion
Metoclopramide (Reglan)	Extrapyramidal effects

Abbreviations: CNS, central nervous system; GI, gastrointestinal; NSAID, nonsteroidal antiinflammatory drug.

Although rounding may be simultaneous or separate, the care provided by the multidisciplinary team requires direction and coordination. The composition of the multidisciplinary team may include surgery, geriatrics, hospital medicine, social work, physical therapy, occupational therapy, nutrition, pharmacy, and discharge planners/use management. Existing hospital care models that exemplify this geriatric-centric strategy include the Hospital Elder Life Program (HELP) and the Acute Care Elderly (ACE) program.[29,30] Daily rounds by this team focus on the geriatric vulnerabilities unique to the elderly and compliment the primary surgical team, which focuses on surgery-specific recovery pathways and avoidance of major morbidity.[31] Advanced care planning is also significantly improved with geriatric consultation, a finding that improved both resource use and bereavement outcomes for families.[32–35]

Function Preservation

Hospitalization is associated with a decline in functional status for older patients, with the odds increasing significantly as patients grow older.[36] For surgical patients, up to 50% of patients do not regain their baseline functional status even at 6 months after discharge.[37] Limited ambulation during the hospital stay has been associated with loss of independent ambulation in older patients.[38] To avoid this decline, early ambulation by nurse-driven or physical therapy protocols has been shown to improve functional status at the time of discharge, and to decrease the likelihood of discharge to a skilled nursing facility.[39–41] Early mobilization is also a key component of enhanced recovery protocols for abdominal surgery, reducing length of stay and cost.[42] Even more important, improving mobility avoids other preventable complications, such as inpatient falls and pressure ulcers, that prolong hospitalization with significant morbidity.[43]

Delirium Prevention

Delirium is an acute change in cognitive status that represents the most common postoperative complication in hospitalized older adults, presenting in up to 60% of older patients.[44] Some risk factors for delirium are inherent to the perioperative process, including sensory and sleep deprivation, polypharmacy, and use of psychoactive drugs. Developing delirium during hospitalization is associated with increased morbidity, mortality, and need for posthospital institutionalization.[45,46]

The cause and thus prevention of delirium is multifactorial (**Table 2**). Interventions to prevent delirium include bedside supportive protocols to maintain orientation, mobilization, sleep hygiene, and sensory deficit support. A common threshold to order the delirium prevention order set is for all patients 75 years of age and older undergoing an inpatient operation, because increasing age is associated with development of delirium.[44] Targeting this population to start a delirium prevention program allows the nursing staff to focus their efforts on a limited truly high-risk population of inpatients. Of note, the evidence currently does not support the belief that prophylactic use of antipsychotics prevents delirium.[47]

Identification and treatment may help decrease the duration of delirium. Screening should be initiated on high-risk patients by a validated tool.[48] As recommended by the American Geriatric Society, first-line therapy for delirious old patients is a multicomponent, nonpharmacologic intervention including (1) frequent orientation, (2) calm environment, (3) eliminated restraint use, (4) familiar objects, and (5) ensuring the use of assistive devices. When patients are at risk to themselves or others, antipsychotics may be used at the lowest effective dose.

Table 2
Modifiable causes of postoperative delirium

Delirium Promotor	Management Strategy
Disorientation	Orient to person, place, time 3 times daily minimum Encourage family presence at bedside
Disrupted sleep	Sleep hygiene: awake during daytime, uninterrupted sleep overnight Windows allowing natural light in room
Immobility	Early ambulation: walk in hallway minimum 3 times daily Avoid tethers: minimize catheters, tubes, lines that discourage walking
Sensory deficits	Vision: wear glasses Hearing: hearing aids/pocket talker
Uncontrolled pain	Nonpharmacologic pain adjuvants (eg, ice, massage) Opioid-sparing multimodal pharmacologic pain management
Medications	Avoid anticholinergic medications and Beers list medications Avoid starting multiple new medications simultaneously
Infection	Avoid iatrogenic infections Diagnose source and actively treat infections

Other Important but Less Common Drivers of Delirium		
• Hypotension	• Hypoxia	• Urinary retention
• Acute blood loss anemia	• Hypercarbia	• Constipation
• Myocardial infarction	• Pulmonary embolus	• Stroke
• Postictal state	• Underhydration	• Malnutrition
• Abnormal sodium level	• Metabolic acidosis	

Appropriate Medication Usage

Medications are another major source of adverse events in hospitalized older adults. Older patients are more sensitive to the effects of benzodiazepines and opioids, in particular, because of a decrease in the number of receptors or affinity of receptors for neurotransmitters.[49] Aging causes a decrease in cardiac output, hepatic and renal outflow, as well as overall decrease in lean body mass with increase in fat that causes redistribution of all drugs and interferes with overall metabolism and clearance.[50] Multiple medications, a phenomenon termed polypharmacy, is both common and deleterious because of drug-drug interactions. For example, starting 5 new medications puts older adults at a 5-fold delirium risk. The Beers list is a medication list considered the gold standard reference for pointing out which medications to avoid in older adults.[51] **Table 1** reviews a subset of medications from the Beers list that are relevant to the perioperative setting.

Postoperative pain control should include multimodal opioid-sparing pain regimens.[7] These pain regimens should include ice packs, massage, standing acetaminophen (1000 mg 3 times a day), gabapentin (300 mg daily), liberal use of regional blocks, and opioids. Appropriate assessment of pain should be made, including using modified pain scales for patients with underlying dementia.[52] Uncontrolled pain has an equal if not greater risk of causing delirium compared with the use of opioids; therefore, opioid use is superior to leaving an older adult with uncontrolled pain.

Nutrition and Hydration

Initiation of nutrition in the postoperative setting should be as expeditious as possible. Swallowing should be evaluated to prevent aspiration, and older patients should be maintained on aspiration precautions while eating.[7] Similar to visual and hearing aids, dentures should be returned as soon as possible. Inclusion of a nutritional supplementation beverage with meals is a common strategy to increase postoperative caloric intake. Ongoing evaluation of adequate food intake should occur throughout the hospital stay.

POSTDISCHARGE CARE OF OLDER ADULTS

Older adults' physiosocial vulnerability makes them uniquely vulnerable to hospital readmission and other adverse outcomes postdischarge. One-third of Medicare patients who had been discharged from the hospital were readmitted within 90 days and more than 50% of patients discharged after surgical procedures were rehospitalized or died within the first year of discharge.[53] Core issues include a poor understanding of what happened during the hospital stay, noncompliance with discharge medical regimen, and a lack of communication with outpatient primary care providers.[29] Optimizing safe discharge practices requires:

Clear discharge instructions: clear review of discharge medical instructions with particular attention paid to newly prescribed medications.

Written instructions: written documents reviewing hospital course and potential postdischarge adverse events such as the occurrence of potential geriatric syndromes, including delirium and falls.

Communication: written communication sent to the older adult's outpatient primary care providers including operation performed and postoperative course, as well as laboratory and diagnostic test results.

Follow-up: prearranged follow-up with surgical team, primary care provider, and any new consultants relevant to inpatient stay.

SUMMARY

Older adults require perioperative care that recognizes and supports their unique physiologic and social needs. There are multiple ongoing national initiatives designed specifically to improve the health care of older adults. The American College of Surgeons Geriatric Surgery Verification Program is the most directly related program to the concepts covered in this article.[22] This verification program outlines 33 evidence-based standards of care directly intended to optimize and improve the surgical care of older adults. Such programs provide financial value through delirium prevention and avoidance of unnecessary operations as well as societal value by maintaining functional independence. With the demographics of an aging population, surgical care that incorporates geriatric specialty care will be increasingly important to achieving the highest quality of surgical care for the population of the United States.

CLINIC CARE POINTS

- Establishing patient-centered treatment goals in surgical therapy revolving around the extension of the patient's healthspan rather than just the consideration of the patient's lifespan is recommended.[2]
- Older patients experience an enhanced morbidity and mortality caused by a multifactorial combination of chronic disease and functional decline.[4]

- The syndrome of frailty represents a distinct vulnerability in older patients. Frailty stratifies risk better than summing comorbidities.[9]
- Age is an independent predictor of risk. The American College of Surgeons recommends using 75 years as the cutoff for high risk because several studies have shown increased morbidity and mortality independently associated with age.[10]
- Prehabilitation has shown decreased postoperative complications and reduced hospital cost.[10]
- Establishment of a multidisciplinary care team composed of all the stakeholders invested in the care of older adults meeting on a regular basis with the goal for implementing evidence-based best practices is strongly recommended.[7]
- The American College of Surgeons has recently modified its widely used surgical risk calculator to more accurately predict morbidities uniquely associated with geriatric patients.[23]
- Intraoperative care of older adults does not differ substantially from usual care models. However, institution of safeguards to avoid pressure injuries, use of regional anesthetic strategies, and avoidance of high-risk medications are recommended.[24–26]
- Existing hospital care models, such as the HELP and the ACE programs, are readily available for implementation.[29,30]
- Use of the Beers list of high-risk medications to avoid has been shown to have significant benefits.[51]
- Multimodal pain control strategies show benefit through reduction in opioid-first pain management strategies.[7]
- Fifty percent of Medicare patients after a surgical procedure are either rehospitalized or die within the first year after discharge. Strategies to mitigate these dynamics include clear written discharge instructions; 360° communication to all stakeholders, particularly primary care providers; and establishment of concrete follow-up.[29,53]

DISCLOSURE

The authors have nothing to disclose.

REFERENCES

1. Center for Disease Control. National Hospital Discharge Survey: number of All Listed Procedures for Discharges from Short-Stay Hospitals, by Procedure Category and Age: United States. Available at: https://www.cdc.gov/nchs/data/nhds/4procedures/2010pro_numberpercentage.pdf. Accessed July 16, 2020.
2. Robinson TN, Zenilman MA. Frailty and the Surgical Care of the Older Adult. In: Cameron JL, Cameron AM, editors. Current surgical therapy. 2017 Philadelphia: Elsevier. p. 1320–25.
3. Crimmins EM. Lifespan and healthspan: past, present, and promise. Gerontologist 2015;55(6):901–11.
4. Bentrem DJ, Cohen ME, Hynes DM, et al. Identification of specific quality improvement opportunities for the elderly undergoing gastrointestinal surgery. Arch Surg 2009;144(11):1013–20.
5. Kwok AC, Semel ME, Lipsitz SR, et al. The intensity and variation of surgical care at the end of life: a retrospective cohort study. Lancet 2011;378(9800):1408–13.
6. Fried TR, Bradley EH, Towle VR, et al. Understanding the treatment preferences of seriously ill patients. N Engl J Med 2002;346(14):1061–6.

7. Mohanty S, Rosenthal RA, Russell MM, et al. Optimal Perioperative Management of the Geriatric Patient: A Best Practices Guideline from the American College of Surgeons NSQIP and the American Geriatrics Society. J Am Coll Surg 2016; 222(5):930–47.

8. Fleisher LA, Fleischmann KE, Auerbach AD, et al. 2014 ACC/AHA guideline on perioperative cardiovascular evaluation and management of patients undergoing noncardiac surgery: a report of the American College of Cardiology/American Heart Association Task Force on practice guidelines. J Am Coll Cardiol 2014; 64(22):e77–137.

9. Rockwood K, Song X, MacKnight C, et al. A global clinical measure of fitness and frailty in elderly people. CMAJ 2005;173(5):489–95.

10. Hamel MB, Henderson WG, Khuri SF, et al. Surgical outcomes for patients aged 80 and older: morbidity and mortality from major noncardiac surgery. J Am Geriatr Soc 2005;53(3):424–9.

11. Plassman BL, Langa KM, Fisher GG, et al. Prevalence of dementia in the United States: the aging, demographics, and memory study. Neuroepidemiology 2007; 29(1-2):125–32.

12. Hu CJ, Liao CC, Chang CC, et al. Postoperative adverse outcomes in surgical patients with dementia: a retrospective cohort study. World J Surg 2012;36(9): 2051–8.

13. Borson S, Scanlan JM, Chen P, et al. The Mini-Cog as a screen for dementia: validation in a population-based sample. J Am Geriatr Soc 2003;51(10):1451–4.

14. Robinson TN, Wu DS, Sauaia A, et al. Slower walking speed forecasts increased postoperative morbidity and 1-year mortality across surgical specialties. Ann Surg 2013;258(4):582–8 [discussion: 588–90].

15. Jones TS, Dunn CL, Wu DS, et al. Relationship between asking an older adult about falls and surgical outcomes. JAMA Surg 2013;148(12):1132–8.

16. Berian JR, Zhou L, Hornor MA, et al. Optimizing surgical quality datasets to care for older adults: Lessons from the American College of Surgeons NSQIP geriatric surgery pilot. J Am Coll Surg 2017;225(6):702–12.e1.

17. Mayo NE, Feldman L, Scott S, et al. Impact of preoperative change in physical function on postoperative recovery: argument supporting prehabilitation for colorectal surgery. Surgery 2011;150(3):505–14.

18. Englesbe MJ, Grenda Dr, Sullivan JA, et al. The Michigan Surgical Home and Optimization Program is a scalable model to improve care and reduce costs. Surgery 2017;161(6):1659–66.

19. Kaiser MJ, et al. Frequency of malnutrition in older adults: a multinational perspective using the mini nutritional assessment. J Am Geriatr Soc 2010; 58(9):1734–8.

20. Herrmann FR, Safran C, Levkoff SE, et al. Serum albumin level on admission as a predictor of death, length of stay, and readmission. Arch Intern Med 1992;152(1): 125–30.

21. Carli F, Bousquet-Dioin G, Awasthi R, et al. Effect of multimodal prehabilitation vs postoperative rehabilitation on 30-day postoperative complications for frail patients undergoing resection of colorectal cancer: a randomized clinical trial. JAMA Surg 2020;155(3):233–42.

22. The American College of Surgeons Geriatric Surgery Verification Quality Improvement Program: Optimal Resources for Geriatric Surgery. Chicago IL: American College of Surgeons; 2019.

23. NSQIP, A. ACS NSQIP surgical risk calculator. 2019. Available at: https:// riskcalculator.facs.org/RiskCalculator/. Accessed July 16, 2020.

24. Nixon J, Cranny G, Bond S. Skin alterations of intact skin and risk factors associated with pressure ulcer development in surgical patients: a cohort study. Int J Nurs Stud 2007;44(5):655–63.

25. Chen DX, Yang L, Ding L, et al. Perioperative outcomes in geriatric patients undergoing hip fracture surgery with different anesthesia techniques: A systematic review and meta-analysis. Medicine (Baltimore) 2019;98(49):e18220.

26. Memtsoudis SG, Poeran J, Zubizarreta N, et al. Do hospitals performing frequent neuraxial anesthesia for hip and knee replacements have better outcomes? Anesthesiology 2018;129(3):428–39.

27. Kristensen PK, Thilemann TM, Soballe K, et al. Can improved quality of care explain the success of orthogeriatric units? A population-based cohort study. Age Ageing 2016;45(1):66–71.

28. Folbert EC, Smit RS, vsn der Velde D, et al. Geriatric fracture center: a multidisciplinary treatment approach for older patients with a hip fracture improved quality of clinical care and short-term treatment outcomes. Geriatr Orthop Surg Rehabil 2012;3(2):59–67.

29. Counsell SR, Holder CM, Liebenauer LL, et al. Effects of a multicomponent intervention on functional outcomes and process of care in hospitalized older patients: a randomized controlled trial of Acute Care for Elders (ACE) in a community hospital. J Am Geriatr Soc 2000;48(12):1572–81.

30. Inouye SK, Bogardus ST, Baker DI, et al. The Hospital Elder Life Program: a model of care to prevent cognitive and functional decline in older hospitalized patients. Hospital Elder Life Program. J Am Geriatr Soc 2000;48(12):1697–706.

31. Chen CC, Lin MT, Tien YW, et al. Modified hospital elder life program: effects on abdominal surgery patients. J Am Coll Surg 2011;213(2):245–52.

32. Fallon WF Jr, Rader E, Zyzanski S, et al. Geriatric outcomes are improved by a geriatric trauma consultation service. J Trauma 2006;61(5):1040–6.

33. Olufajo OA, Tulebaev S, Javedan H, et al. Integrating geriatric consults into routine care of older trauma patients: one-year experience of a level i trauma center. J Am Coll Surg 2016;222(6):1029–35.

34. Zhang B, Wright AA, Huskamp HA, et al. Health care costs in the last week of life: associations with end-of-life conversations. Arch Intern Med 2009;169(5):480–8.

35. Greer JA, Pirl WF, Jackson VA, et al. Effect of early palliative care on chemotherapy use and end-of-life care in patients with metastatic non-small-cell lung cancer. J Clin Oncol 2012;30(4):394–400.

36. Covinsky KE, Palmer RM, Fortinsky RH, et al. Loss of independence in activities of daily living in older adults hospitalized with medical illnesses: increased vulnerability with age. J Am Geriatr Soc 2003;51(4):451–8.

37. Lawrence VA, Hazuda HP, Cornell JE, et al. Functional independence after major abdominal surgery in the elderly. J Am Coll Surg 2004;199(5):762–72.

38. Callahan EH, Thomas DC, Goldhirsch SL, et al. Geriatric hospital medicine. Med Clin North Am 2002;86(4):707–29.

39. Padula CA, Hughes C, Baumhover L. Impact of a nurse-driven mobility protocol on functional decline in hospitalized older adults. J Nurs Care Qual 2009;24(4):325–31.

40. King BJ, Steege LM, Winsor K, et al. Getting patients walking: a pilot study of mobilizing older adult patients via a nurse-driven intervention. J Am Geriatr Soc 2016;64(10):2088–94.

41. Hastings SN, Sloane R, Morey M, et al. Assisted early mobility for hospitalized older veterans: preliminary data from the STRIDE program. J Am Geriatr Soc 2014;62(11):2180–4.

42. Bond-Smith G, Belgaumkar AP, Davidson BR, et al. Enhanced recovery protocols for major upper gastrointestinal, liver and pancreatic surgery. Cochrane Database Syst Rev 2016;(2):CD011382.

43. Lane AJ. Evaluation of the fall prevention program in an acute care setting. Orthop Nurs 1999;18(6):37–43.

44. Siddiqi N, Harrison JK, Clegg A, et al. Interventions for preventing delirium in hospitalised non-ICU patients. Cochrane Database Syst Rev 2016;(3):Cd005563.

45. Demeure MJ, Fain MJ. The elderly surgical patient and postoperative delirium. J Am Coll Surg 2006;203(5):752–7.

46. Witlox J, Eurelings LS, de Jonghe JF, et al. Delirium in elderly patients and the risk of postdischarge mortality, institutionalization, and dementia: a meta-analysis. JAMA 2010;304(4):443–51.

47. Oh ES, Needham DM, Nikooie R, et al. Antipsychotics for preventing delirium in hospitalized adults: a systematic review. Ann Intern Med 2019;171(7):474–84.

48. Society AG. AGES Expert Panel on postoperative delirium in older adults. American geriatrics society clinical practice guideline for postoperative delirium in older adults. 2014. Available at: https://geriatricscareonline.org/toc/american-geriatrics-society-clinical-practice-guideline-for-postoperative-delirium-in-older-adults/CL018/. Accessed July 16, 2020.

49. Feely J, Coakley D. Altered pharmacodynamics in the elderly. Clin Geriatr Med 1990;6(2):269–83.

50. Muravchick S. Anesthesia for the elderly. In: Miller RD, editor. Anesthesia. New York: Churchill Livingstone; 1994. p. 2143–56.

51. American Geriatrics Society 2019 Updated AGS Beers Criteria(R) for Potentially Inappropriate Medication Use in Older Adults. J Am Geriatr Soc 2019;67(4):674–94.

52. Malara A, De Biase GA, Bettarini F, et al. Pain Assessment in Elderly with Behavioral and Psychological Symptoms of Dementia. J Alzheimers Dis 2016;50(4):1217–25.

53. Jencks SF, Williams MV, Coleman EA. Rehospitalizations among patients in the Medicare fee-for-service program. N Engl J Med 2009;360(14):1418–28.

Challenges Related to Safety and Independence

Hannah Ward, MD[a], Thomas E. Finucane, MD[b], Mattan Schuchman, MD[c],*

KEYWORDS

- Geriatrics • Older adults • Autonomy • Risk • Independence • Safety • Ethics

KEY POINTS

- Perceptions of safety and risk vary widely, throughout society and among clinicians and patients.
- When safety and independence are in conflict, clinicians should consider several factors: the patient's perspective, the perspectives of other major stakeholders, the magnitude of patient risk and risk to others, clinician biases, and liability.
- The goal in general is not to find the right answer, but to find a fair, transparent way to choose among morally acceptable alternatives, fashioning a consensus agreement on a strategy that optimizes both safety and independence.
- When a patient's civil liberties might be abridged, involvement of the state may be necessary.

CLINICAL CASES

Case 1

Ms J is a 68-year-old who is seen in the office for routine primary care follow-up. Her medical conditions include rheumatoid arthritis and advanced chronic obstructive pulmonary disease. She has significant joint destruction in her hands and feet. She requires supplemental oxygen and is dyspneic with any exertion. She uses a wheelchair for mobility and requires assistance for most of her activities of daily living. She lives with her husband who is also her caregiver. Her husband works outside the home during the day, during which time Ms J is often alone. During the visit, her primary care physician notes poor personal hygiene and multiple pressure injuries and wounds. A recent note in her chart from the home-health registered nurse says the home is unfit for habitation and that Ms J is home alone in soiled clothing, with no way to call for help. Ms J's physician is concerned that her recurrent skin infections and wounds, which have led to several hospitalizations, are related to inadequate

[a] Department of Internal Medicine, Johns Hopkins Bayview Medical Center, 4940 Eastern Avenue, 3rd Floor, Baltimore, MD 21224, USA; [b] Harvard Medical School, Massachusetts General Hospital, 165 Cambridge Street., Senior Health, 5th Floor, Boston, MA 02114, USA; [c] Division of Geriatric Medicine and Gerontology, Johns Hopkins University School of Medicine, Mason F. Lord Building - Suite 2200, 5200 Eastern Avenue, Baltimore, MD 21224, USA
* Corresponding author.
E-mail address: mattan@jhmi.edu

Med Clin N Am 104 (2020) 909–917
https://doi.org/10.1016/j.mcna.2020.06.006
0025-7125/20/© 2020 Elsevier Inc. All rights reserved.

care. She was previously admitted to a skilled nursing facility after a hospitalization but left against medical advice because she felt frustrated with her care there. She adamantly refuses to return to any facility. She acknowledges that her current situation is not ideal and requests help finding additional caregiving resources and help with improving the home condition. Despite knowing that these services are not immediately available to her, Ms J wants to remain in her current home.

Case 2

You receive a call from the neighbor of your patient, Mr L, informing you that Mr L had another fall. The neighbor says that Mr L was walking toward Maple Avenue, a busy street, at 5 AM and not wearing a coat despite the freezing weather. The neighbor found him having fallen on an uneven lawn. Mr L says he was going to a fast food place to get dinner but did not realize the place was not yet open. He thought it was 5 PM rather than 5 AM. Mr L lives alone in the house where he was born 85 years ago. His neighbor checks in on him every day, brings over groceries, and does small errands. Mr L used to rely on his nephew, but the nephew formally resigned as his power of attorney out of frustration because Mr L refused to move, hire an aide, or modify his living situation. Mr L would call the nephew up to 15 times a night with repetitive questions. You do a house call for Mr L and see that belongings are piling up. There is a strong odor. It is clear that he is sleeping in his recliner rather than his bed upstairs. He takes none of the medications that you had prescribed for coronary artery disease. You gently engage him in a conversation about his care, and when you say assisted living facility he says "No! No! No!"

Case 3

Ms F is an avid bingo player. She is a widow and drives to the bingo hall each week to see her friends, an outing that is the center of her social life. She has been living with diabetes for many years. In the last few years, the neuropathy in her legs has worsened and is now also affecting her fingers. Over the past year, she has had 3 fender-benders in which she knocked over a neighbor's mailbox, scraped her garage wall, and had a minor parking lot collision. For the past year, her 2 daughters have forbidden her grandchildren from riding in the car with her. On examination, she has diminished awareness of joint positioning and a loss of sensation to light touch in both her feet and ankles. When you bring up concern about her driving, she immediately gets defensive: "I only drive during the day, I go slowly, and I stay in my neighborhood on roads that I know like the back of my hand." Despite her protest, you make a firm recommendation that she no longer drive and ask a community health worker to meet with Ms F to see whether there are other ways that she could still get to bingo.

INTRODUCTION

Balancing safety and independence is a fundamental challenge for most humans. The balancing act can be seen in sharpest relief at the extremes of age: in childhood, adolescence, and old age. Need for substitute decision makers and the involvement of the state can affect how the balance is achieved. In 2015, the parents of a 6-year-old and a 10-year-old were charged with child neglect for allowing their children to walk home alone from neighborhood playgrounds in the suburbs of Washington, DC. The parents were ultimately cleared of charges, but the debate was furious.[1] Did the risk to which these parents exposed their children amount to criminal disregard for safety? On a larger scale, in 1919 the 18th Amendment ushering in prohibition was ratified in 46 of 48 states and became the law of the land for more than a decade. Although an element of moral judgment contributed to the amendment's passage, improved public health was a central argument. Rates of alcoholism, cirrhosis, and death from cirrhosis decreased sharply. Prohibition ended with the 21st Amendment, and "an excess of 13,665 infant deaths ... could be attributable to the repeal of federal prohibition in 1933."[2] Reestablishing prohibition now seems inconceivable.

Four factors ensure that these debates often defy a simple resolution. First, it is rarely possible to provide a precise quantitative assessment of risk. For example, what is the risk of staying home alone in squalid conditions, as in cases 1 and 2? Who defines what squalid means? Second, even if a precise quantitative statement of risk were possible, there is no societal agreement on what is too risky. Third, the ability to make a meaningful decision (in medical terms, capacity) about a known level of risk can vary over time. Fourth, American society, with its emphasis on individualism, is far from achieving a stable consensus on the role of the state or medical authority in regulating risks.

Decisions that balance maintenance of independence with promotion of safety frequently challenge older adults and their health care providers. These challenges commonly arise in decisions about living environment and driving and, as such, may include both social and medical factors. From physical rehabilitation to the installation of home modifications to a change of residence (with a change in level of care), many decisions about health care for vulnerable older adults focus on safety. Several factors combine to make the challenges particularly complex. As adults age, rates of frailty, medical illness, and disability increase, increasing the risk of everyday behaviors. Factors that help to mitigate risk, such as social networks and financial resources, may dwindle. Cognitive dysfunction may decrease an individual's ability to assess risk accurately and make sound decisions. Each of these factors may be progressive.

This article is intended to help clinicians working with older adults navigate challenges to safety and independence. It begins with a brief discussion of clinicians' ethical obligations toward patients and how these obligations ground their approach to negotiating safety and independence. It presents safety and risk as inherently subjective clinical assessments for which there is no gold standard measurement. It then considers several factors that may help clinicians when assessing safety challenges in the care of individual patients, including evaluation of decision-making capacity. It suggests some pragmatic strategies for addressing these challenges in commonly encountered clinical scenarios, such as the cases at the beginning of this article.

DISCUSSION
Ethical Obligations to Patients

Clinicians have an ethical obligation to promote their patients' health and prevent harm. These duties arise from the principles of beneficence and nonmaleficence. However, clinicians' ethical obligations are not limited to these fundamental principles. Beauchamp and Childress's[3] now-classic formulation of bioethics puts equal or greater weight on patient autonomy. In some situations, such as cases 1 and 2, in which a patient desires to live at home despite high risk and even actual harms, these ethical obligations, to promote health and prevent harm on one hand and to respect the patient's self-determination on the other, may be at odds.[4] Clinicians are also constrained by the requirement of nonabandonment, the commitment that clinicians make to remain with the patients, to continue to work with them, and to face an uncertain future together without necessarily agreeing with the patients' decisions.[5]

Safety and Risk

In most clinical scenarios, clinicians cannot objectively measure risk, but must instead estimate it based on experience, published data, or both. Validated tools exist to estimate certain risks. In other cases, individuals must rely on their life experience and the professional judgment of physicians, physical therapists, or other health care providers. A patient may have an increased risk of falling based on a validated tool and clinical assessment, but whether moving from home to an assisted living facility will reduce the risk of a complex multifactorial outcome such as a hip fracture is not knowable.

Patients may engage in high-risk activities, such as continuing to drive or to live alone, because they assume that their doctors would have told them if their behaviors were unsafe.[6] Although clinicians often primarily consider physical safety, this is only 1 aspect of what may be important to a patient or caregiver. Patients with full knowledge and full capacity may choose to accept high levels of physical risk for a host of factors, including emotional safety, financial safety, integrity, dignity, privacy, and personal relationships. Clinician and patient should work together to identify and clarify the patient's values and priorities in order to facilitate sound decision making. If a given high-risk behavior aligns with a patient's stated values, the decision to accept this risk is more clearly justified. For example, if a patient places high value on remaining (and dying) in the patient's lifelong home, a place that is associated with familial relationships and safety, then the patient may accept substantial risks in order to achieve that goal. Furthermore, a patient in this scenario may not be as concerned with the risk of death and instead may be focused on the risks of pain or discomfort. Understanding motivation helps clinicians support people to make authentic personal choices rather than choices that optimize only physical safety from a medical standpoint.

Clinical Approach

Box 1 lists several of the factors that should be made as transparent as possible to all who are part of the decision-making process when facing a situation in which there is a challenge to safety and independence.

Magnitude of risk

Estimating risk requires making predictions about the future. For many patients and their loved ones, probability and the quickly branching chains of various hypothetical outcomes are extremely difficult tools to use in decision making. Online tools provide visual aids that may help in conceptualizing risk of mortality or other adverse outcomes in some situations.[7] Providing written material to the patients can be helpful for both the patients and their companions, who may not retain all a clinician says, and for loved ones who were not at the meeting.

Box 1
Recommended factors for clinicians to consider when assessing potentially unsafe choices

- Magnitude of risk: what are the likelihood and severity of potential adverse outcomes? Is there risk to others? Do I understand what risks most concern this patient?

- Decision-making capacity: does this patient understand relevant details, benefits, burdens, and alternatives?

- Collateral information: with the patient's permission, have I elicited the perspectives of friends and family?

- Clinician bias: how do my values and life experiences shape and bias my assessment of safety?

- Alternatives: what compromises or risk-mitigating strategies are available?

- Liability: are there legal or professional requirements that I must fulfill?

Risk to others is a separate consideration, distinct from risk to self. For example, continuing to drive despite demonstrably increased risk of doing so (for various reasons, including declining vision, reflexes, judgment, substance abuse, peripheral neuropathy, or epilepsy) endangers not only the driver but also the public, as in case 3. In most jurisdictions, risk to others at certain thresholds supersedes autonomy of a competent individual. Some states (eg, California, Pennsylvania, and New Jersey) require that providers report their medically or cognitively impaired patients to the Department of Motor Vehicles. Analogously, reporting to the Department of Health is mandatory for infectious diseases such as tuberculosis or syphilis. Sometimes, if a clinician detects credible risk of harm to others, the clinician must override a person's autonomy, compromise privacy, and hospitalize the person involuntarily through the courts and law enforcement. Reporting patients who are immediate threats to others is widely permitted in some circumstances, such as imminent threats of violence to others. However, there is considerable gray area in between what constitutes an obvious danger and a low level of risk.

Decision-making capacity

A patient's capacity to make a meaningful decision significantly changes the appropriate course of action. The threshold for capacity changes relative to the risk. For situations where risk is high, the scrutiny of an individual's capacity is greater. Although clinician judgments about capacity may vary along this spectrum, clinicians are often asked to make a yes-or-no judgment. No formulaic test can prove presence or absence of capacity; the assessment of capacity requires a discussion with the patient. **Box 2** lists several questions that may be useful to clinicians during such a discussion. These questions also help clinicians understand how patients' values are informing their choices and their risk tolerance.

When a clinician determines that a patient lacks capacity, there should still be an attempt made to incorporate the patient's current or previously stated preferences and show respect for the person into decisions made on the person's behalf. When accepting risk for patients who lack capacity, clinicians and caregivers should try to mitigate any potential harms that may accompany the patient's wishes. Respect for current and previously expressed preferences is important but may not be decisive and may not always be possible.

If a substitute decision maker is needed for a specific decision, the patient may retain the ability to make other decisions. For example, because of safety concerns, a person may be required to move from independent living to assisted living despite wishing to remain at home. That person might still participate in choosing the facility that will become home.

For a patient with diminished capacity, decisions that focus only on decreasing risk and increasing safety may undermine the patient's dignity. This concept, the dignity of risk, was introduced in 1972 by Robert Perske,[8] an advocate for people with

---

Box 2
Example questions to use in discussions assessing capacity

Tell me in your own words what decision you are considering.

What are some possible upsides and downsides of that choice?

What other options might you have?

Why are you choosing option A instead of option B?

intellectual and developmental disabilities (IDDs).He noted that, among people with IDDs, denying any risk "tends to have a deleterious effect on both their sense of human dignity and their personal development. In addition, the removal of all risk diminishes the retarded [sic] in the eyes of others."[8] The same is likely true for the elderly.[9] Despite clinicians' best intentions, they may cause harm when they focus too narrowly on physical safety.

When a patient has diminished capacity, risk levels are extremely high, and no compromise strategy can be found, outside intervention may be required. This major escalation can generate great burden for all concerned, but due-process safeguards are necessary when a person may lose fundamental civil liberties. The legal steps vary from state to state and may involve Adult Protective Services, emergency petition, and guardianship. Alternatives to guardianship, which seek ways to balance independence and safety with nonadversarial approaches that still provide due process of law, are under study.[10] It is rare, but possible, for individuals to argue that they have regained capacity and formally regain independence and an end to guardianship.

Laws and nomenclature about substitute decision makers (SDMs) vary widely by jurisdiction, creating potential confusion for clinicians, patients, families, and support systems. A person could be acting as an SDM because the patient assigned this role, or by default as next of kin. Although designated and default SDMs hold comparable levels of authority in some jurisdictions, in others the designated SDM has significantly more authority than the default SDM. The terminology for designated and default SDMs varies widely by jurisdiction. Many states refer to designated SDMs as health care agents or durable powers of attorney. Some states use the terms proxy or surrogate to refer to default decision makers, but the same terms may refer to the designated SDM or simply any SDM in another state. In sum, the authority of an SDM to guide the treatment of a patient depends heavily on the regulations of the local jurisdiction.

Perspective of family and friends

Involvement of a patient's family or support network is often critical and, when possible, should only be done with the patient's permission. It is helpful to ask a patient, "Is there anyone else who may be affected by this decision with whom we should talk?" The ultimate decision remains that of the patient or, when decision capacity is lacking, a surrogate decision maker (or makers).

Inviting the perspective of the family and support network helps put an individual's decisions into context, can be helpful in capacity determination, and can generate a more durable solution because it is supported by friends and family. Impact on others may drive an individual's motivation for one choice or another. Older adults often fear being a burden on others.[11] Having the support network engaged in the conversation can thus help patients clarify assumptions about their impact on their caregivers and loved ones, whose perspectives may differ greatly from what the patient anticipates. Consider what hypothetical adult children might think if they perceive their loved ones to be in a high-risk situation (**Box 3**). In some situations, the clinician may have to explain to the loved ones that the patient is able to make decisions that caregivers would consider unsafe, whereas, in other cases, collateral information from caregivers makes it evident that a person lacks decision-making capacity. Adult children face very difficult choices when their frail parents insist on choosing risky options. The caregivers may wish to ally with the clinician to tell their loved one what to do (eg, "Doc, you have to tell Mom to stop doing…"). In these cases, clinicians need to be sure to make an independent assessment of the situation.

> **Box 3**
> **What the adult child might be thinking**
>
> I can't bear the thought of my mom with a new serious injury.
>
> I couldn't live with it if she is badly harmed and I said "OK."
>
> What will my siblings/partner/neighbors say?
>
> I can't let this happen.
>
> I can't keep doing this for much longer.

Clinician bias

Clinicians' ability to accurately assess risk and judge capacity is subject to bias. Awareness of personal biases is therefore critical for reducing their impact. Biases can include notions about what is appropriate for persons based on their age, gender, race, socioeconomic status, cognitive and physical ability, and somatic and psychiatric health conditions. Ageism and ableism may lead clinicians to overestimate risk. Clinicians' cultural expectations, lived experience, and values shape perceptions of risk. For example, poor hygiene is a commonly cited risk factor for development of skin and wound infections. Poor hygiene is a subjective determination and the evidence supporting this belief is equivocal and limited.[12] An older adult initiating a new sexual relationship is another example. This relationship can be profoundly disturbing to relatives, who may couch their objection as a safety issue.

Deviation from dominant cultural norms of dressing, hygiene, or social behavior may serve as triggers for clinicians and social workers to assess the safety of individuals in their current situations. The authors suggest that clinicians carefully scrutinize such concerns before taking action. Is there truly a safety issue at heart? Changes in personal hygiene or housekeeping may alert clinicians to a developing medical disorder such as dementia or depression, but deviations from social norms may also simply reflect personal and social variation or an accommodation to difficult circumstances. Distinguishing among these requires clinician self-awareness. Collateral information from loved ones can be particularly informative in these situations. It is not the job of clinicians, nor is it ethical, to enforce a bourgeois lifestyle or impose their personal standard of living on their patients.

Considering questions such as those in **Box 4** may help clinicians reflect on their own values and views informing safety and risk. Importantly, awareness of personal biases is lifelong work. The authors encourage clinicians to revisit this topic periodically. The goals and values of an 80-year-old, or of a caregiving 45-year-old adult child, may not be intuitively obvious to a 35-year-old medical professional.

Alternatives: making the best of it

If a person chooses to remain in a risky situation at home, harm reduction strategies include home safety upgrades, home monitoring devices, and increased frequency of

> **Box 4**
> **Empathy in difficult situations: the do-unto-others test**
>
> What are some choices that I have made that put myself or others at risk?
>
> How much personal surveillance would I be OK with?
>
> What would I consider an acceptable standard of living?
>
> How much risk, inconvenience, and reduced hygiene would I accept in order to stay at home rather than entering a nursing home?

check-ins by family members or professional caregivers. Widely available community resources include meal delivery services, paid caregiver services, and mobility services such as senior rides. Other supports may be available. All states have Medicaid waiver programs of various forms and availabilities to help provide low-income patients with in-home support.

These risk mitigation strategies may themselves be unacceptable to patients. Patients may perceive home monitoring devices such as cameras or fall detection systems as intrusive.[13] Older adults may not see the value of spending the money, or have the money available, to afford in-home aides, who may seem intrusive to patients. Clinicians should revisit these strategies periodically with patients and their loved ones, because changes in conditions may lead to reconsideration of priorities.

Considering liability

Clinicians may be concerned about liability if a patient makes an unsafe choice. In certain situations, clinicians are legally required to report concerns for abuse, financial exploitation, neglect, or self-neglect perpetrated against vulnerable adults, especially those who have significant cognitive impairment. It is important to be aware of the laws of the local jurisdiction. Documentation in the medical record is important both for potential liability issues and to clarify for other clinicians the process by which the current circumstances were fashioned. This record-keeping avoids the unnecessary repetition of conversations that are often burdensome to all concerned.

The practices of dismissing patients from a clinic practice, ending the doctor-patient relationship, and of discharging patients from a hospital or other care facility against medical advice may sometimes be considered when caring for patients whose disregard for the safety of self or others exceeds some important threshold. These complex topics are not considered here, in part because there are considerable legal and policy dimensions to each of these practices.

SUMMARY

The cases presented at the beginning of this article feature patients who choose to live at home and to drive, despite health care providers' concerns about the significant risks of doing so. These cases are examples in which older adults, their families, and their clinicians must balance risk reduction with autonomy and respect for person. To further complicate such decisions, there is significant ambiguity regarding risk, both in how much risk a decision entails and in how much risk is too much. Capacity to make a given decision may vary over time, and the authority of surrogate decision makers varies between jurisdictions. Clinicians should seek to understand the patient's (and, with permission, other relevant parties') perspectives, and should be mindful of how their own biases may affect their assessment of a situation. In cases where there is significant risk to others, or when a vulnerable patient is in a high-risk situation, outside intervention may be needed. In other situations, clinicians should partner with patients and their families to be transparent about the decision-making process and to find ways to reduce risk that all parties deem acceptable. In all cases, the goal is to support the patient in making choices that are authentic to their values and preferences.

CLINICAL CARE POINTS

- Risk is often difficult to quantify; communicating it clearly and accurately to patients is often even more difficult. Written and visual materials can be helpful to complement verbal communication.

- Evaluation of capacity to make a decision requires a discussion with the patient, rather than reliance on tools or formulaic tests. Capacity may vary continuously and fluctuate over time.
- Risk mitigation strategies include using community resources, paid caregivers, and technology such as surveillance devices. These strategies are not accessible or acceptable to all patients, and some may find them intrusive.
- Situations in which there is significant risk to others, or in which a vulnerable patient is in a high-risk situation, generally require outside intervention, such as involvement of Adult Protective Services or emergency petition via law enforcement. Specifics of these interventions vary by jurisdiction.

DISCLOSURE

The authors have nothing to disclose.

REFERENCES

1. George St, Donna. 'Free range' parents cleared in second neglect case after kids walked alone. The Washington Post 2015. Available at: https://www.washingtonpost.com/local/education/free-range-parents-cleared-in-second-neglect-case-after-children-walked-alone/2015/06/22/82283c24-188c-11e5-bd7f-4611a60dd8e5_story.html. Accessed February 11 2020.
2. Jacks DS, Pendakur K, Shigeoka H. Infant Mortality and the Repeal of Federal Prohibition," NBER Working Papers 23372, National Bureau of Economic Research, Inc. 2017.
3. Beauchamp TL, Childress JF. Principles of biomedical ethics. 5th edition. New York: Oxford University Press; 2001.
4. Carrese JA. Refusal of care: patients' well-being and physicians' ethical obligations: "But doctor, I want to go home. JAMA 2006;296(6):691–5.
5. Quill TE, Cassel CK. Nonabandonment: a central obligation for physicians. Ann Intern Med 1995;122(5):368–74.
6. Moore LW, Miller M. Driving strategies used by older adults with macular degeneration: assessing the risks. Appl Nurs Res 2005;18(2):110–6.
7. Lee S, Smith A, Widera E, et al. ePrognosis. Available at: https://eprognosis.ucsf.edu/. Accessed February 11 2020.
8. Perske R. The dignity of risk and the mentally retarded. Ment Retard 1972;10(1):24–7.
9. Rush KL, Murphy MA, Kozak JF. A photovoice study of older adults' conceptualizations of risk. J Aging Stud 2012;26(4):448–58.
10. Beyond guardianship: towards alternatives that promote greater self-determination. National Council on Disability; 2018.
11. Bell S, Menec V. "You don't want to ask for the help" the imperative of independence: is it related to social exclusion? J Appl Gerontol 2015;34(3):NP1–21.
12. Barkhuff D, Nitta CH, Cobb R, et al. Bathing habits in emergency department patients with cellulitis or abscess versus controls. South Med J 2018;111(8):489–93.
13. Berridge C, Wetle TF. Why older adults and their children disagree about in-home surveillance technology, sensors, and tracking. Gerontologist 2019. https://doi.org/10.1093/geront/gnz068.

Moving?

Make sure your subscription moves with you!

To notify us of your new address, find your **Clinics Account Number** (located on your mailing label above your name), and contact customer service at:

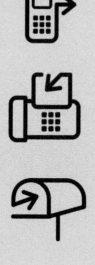

Email: journalscustomerservice-usa@elsevier.com

800-654-2452 (subscribers in the U.S. & Canada)
314-447-8871 (subscribers outside of the U.S. & Canada)

Fax number: 314-447-8029

Elsevier Health Sciences Division
Subscription Customer Service
3251 Riverport Lane
Maryland Heights, MO 63043

*To ensure uninterrupted delivery of your subscription, please notify us at least 4 weeks in advance of move.

Printed and bound by CPI Group (UK) Ltd, Croydon, CR0 4YY

03/10/2024

01040407-0016